The healing bond

The Healing Bond explores the nature of the relationship between healer and patient in a variety of settings, with the emphasis on the issue of therapeutic responsibility. The contributors – health care professionals and social scientists – investigate how responsibility is distributed between healer and patient. Can it be shared among more than one practitioner? What is the role of professional organizations in defining and safeguarding the relationship? Is the bond between the healer and practitioner a dynamic aspect of the healing process itself? If the bond changes over time, what wider social forces influence it?

These questions are investigated from a variety of professional and academic perspectives, covering both 'orthodox' and 'non-orthodox' forms of healing practice. The contributors look at health care as a whole and deal with specific areas of health such as midwifery, psychoanalysis, naturopathy, the relations between medicine and the state, and the appeal of 'quacks'. They also confront particular issues of current concern, including medical litigation, codes of ethics for complementary practitioners, and cooperation between orthodox and complementary medicine.

Written by people from a wide range of backgrounds – medical sociology, anthropology, psychoanalysis, medicine, complementary therapy, the law – *The Healing Bond* is unique in taking into account the perspectives of the healers themselves. It will therefore be of great value to students, teachers and practitioners in a variety of disciplines, including medical sociology, anthropology and medicine, as well as to healers.

Susan Budd, previously a Lecturer in Sociology at the London School of Economics, is a psychoanalyst in private practice. **Ursula Sharma** is a Reader in Sociology and Social Anthropology at the University of Keele.

The healing bond

The patient–practitioner relationship and therapeutic responsibility

Edited by
Susan Budd
and
Ursula Sharma

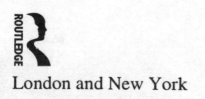

London and New York

First published 1994
by Routledge
11 New Fetter Lane, London EC4P 4EE

Simultaneously published in the USA and Canada
by Routledge
29 West 35th Street, New York, NY 10001

Typeset in Times by LaserScript, Mitcham, Surrey
Printed and bound in Great Britain by
Mackays of Chatham PLC, Chatham, Kent

British Library Cataloguing in Publication Data
A catalogue record for this book is available from the British Library.

Library of Congress Cataloging in Publication Data
The Healing Bond: the patient–practitioner relationship and
therapeutic responsibility/edited by Susan Budd and Ursula Sharma
   p.   cm.
Includes bibliographical references and index.
1. Medical personnel and patient. I. Budd, Susan, 1941–
II. Sharma, Ursula, 1941– .
[DNLM: 1. Physician–Patient Relations. 2. Therapeutics.
3. Ethics, Medical. W 62 H434 1994]
R727.3.H417   1994
610.69′6 – dc20
DNLM/DLC
for Library of Congress
94-990
CIP

ISBN 0–415–09051–2 (hbk)
ISBN 0–415–09052–0 (pbk)

This book is dedicated to the memory of
Om Prakasha Sharma
(1933–1992)
who would have been a healer

Contents

Notes on contributors

Susan Budd graduated in sociology from the London School of Economics where she and Ursula Sharma met. She then went on to Oxford to do the research which was published as *Varieties of Unbelief: Atheists and Agnostics in English Society 1850–1960* (Heinemann Educational Books, 1976). She is also the author of *Sociologists and Religion* (Collier-Macmillan, 1972) and various articles. She returned to the London School of Economics as a lecturer, and became visiting lecturer to the MSc course in Community Medicine at the London School of Hygiene and Tropical Medicine. She then retrained as a psychoanalyst, and is now a member of the British Psychoanalytical Society and works in private practice in London.

Mary Douglas is an anthropologist with African experience and interests. Other longstanding areas of research concern include the methodology of the social sciences, the politicization of nature, rival representations of danger and rival theories of psyche and justice as well as the problem of how to avoid an ethnocentric basis for social thought. After retiring from University College London in 1977 Mary Douglas taught in the United States and is now retired in London. Her main publications include *Purity and Danger* (Routledge, 1966), *Natural Symbols* (Barrie and Rockcliffe, 1970), *Essays in the Sociology of Perception* (Routledge, 1982), *Risk and Culture* (California University Press, 1982), *Risk Acceptability according to the Social Sciences* (Routledge, 1985), *How Institutions Think* (Syracuse University Press, 1986) and *Risk and Blame: Essays in Cultural Theory* (Routledge, 1992).

Calliope Farsides took her doctorate at the London School of Economics and now teaches in the Philosophy Department at Keele University. She is the Director of the Centre for Contemporary Ethical Studies at Keele, where she runs the Diploma and MA courses in Medical Ethics and the Diploma in Ethics of Cancer and Palliative Care. She is a member of the

Local Research Ethics Committee in North Staffordshire and is on the steering committee of the United Kingdom Forum on Health Care Ethics and Law. At present she is engaged in multidisciplinary research funded by the EC on 'Aids, Justice and European Social Policy'.

David Peters is a general practitioner. He trained as a homoeopath after qualifying in medicine in 1972, was a GP trainer in his own NHS practice and a lecturer in the Department of General Practice at St Mary's Paddington for several years before he qualified in osteopathic medicine in 1986 and joined the clinical team at Marylebone Health Centre in London. He practises there and is researching the role of complementary medicine in general practice. He is also Course Director of a new Master's degree in Therapeutic Bodywork.

Roy Porter is Reader in the Social History of Medicine at the Wellcome Institute for the History of Medicine. He is currently working on the history of hysteria. Recent books include *Mind Forg'd Manacles: Madness in England from the Restoration to the Regency* (Athlone, 1987), *A Social History of Madness* (Weidenfeld & Nicholson, 1987), *In Sickness and in Health: The British Experience 1650–1850* (Fourth Estate, 1988), *Patient's Progress: Doctors and Doctoring in Eighteenth-Century England* (Polity, 1989) – these last two being co-authored with Dorothy Porter – and *Health for Sale: Quackery in England 1650–1850* (Manchester University Press, 1989).

Richenda Power is a practising osteopath and naturopath. She has also completed a PhD in sociology, entitled *The Whole Idea: A Critical Evaluation of the Emergence of 'Holistic Medicine' in the Early 1980s*. She does part-time teaching for South Bank University and the Open University, and is currently a member of a working party on research ethics in osteopathy for the General Council and Register of Osteopaths.

Ursula Sharma teaches sociology and social anthropology at Keele University, specializing in medical anthropology. She has carried out research on a number of areas in anthropology, mainly concerned with gender and the household in India on which she has published *Women, Work and Property* (Tavistock, 1980) and *Women's Work, Class and the Urban Household* (Tavistock, 1986). At present she is engaged in long-term research on complementary medicine in Britain, including a project on 'Professionalization in Complementary Medicine'. She is the author of *Complementary Medicine Today: Practitioners and Patients* (Routledge, 1992).

Margaret Stacey is Emeritus Professor of Sociology at Warwick University. She has focused on issues in the sociology of health for the past thirty years, editing *Hospitals, Children and Their Families* (Routledge & Kegan

Paul, 1970) and (with David Hall) *Beyond Separation: Further Studies of Children in Hospital* (Routledge & Kegan Paul, 1979). She is also the author of *Sociology of Health and Healing* (Unwin Hyman, 1988). She has served on the Welsh Hospital Board, the Michael Davies Committee on Hospital Complaints Procedures and, as a lay member, the General Medical Council. From this derives her *Regulating Medicine: The General Medical Council* (Wiley, 1992).

Robert Sumerling has been qualified as a solicitor since 1969. He is a partner in the London legal firm of Le Brasseurs, which has had over a century of experience in the conventional health care field. He has wide experience of advising conventional health providers, that is, NHS trusts, private hospitals and general practitioners. His areas of particular interest include ethical advice and defence of doctors, dentists and midwives in professional conduct cases. He thinks that there should be a synergy rather than an antagonism between conventional and alternative medicine, and so welcomes the chance to explore here the legal and constitutional lessons which each can bring to the other.

Gillian Vanhegan is a gynaecologist who has specialized in psychosexual medicine. She is Medical Director of the London Brook Advisory Centre, which advises young people on contraception and sexual health. Dr Vanhegan is a member of the Institute of Psychosexual Medicine and is its medical research officer.

Introduction

Susan Budd and Ursula Sharma

THE SCOPE OF THIS BOOK

This book is an attempt to explore one of the most important relationships in our lives – that between a person who feels or is told that he or she is sick or ailing in some way, and a person who tries to offer (professional) help.

This help has two components – the diagnostic knowledge and treatment that the expert can offer, and the relationship within which they are offered. Our title, *The Healing Bond*, conveys this double meaning: the relationship between healer and patient not only is a means of delivering treatment but also is, or can be, an aspect of healing itself. Orthodox medicine recognizes this, but focuses on the treatment which is offered by an expert to the patient as a passive recipient. In other forms of treatment the stress may be rather different. In psychoanalysis, for example, and in many forms of alternative medicine, the relationship between the sufferer and the therapist is acknowledged to be a more personal and intimate one, and the conception of treatment lays more explicit stress on the need for patients to participate in their own recovery.

Medical sociologists have studied the healing bond mainly in terms of relationships between patients and orthodox doctors. Much work in this field is informed by a desire to expose and explore the power dimension of this relationship, especially those forms of power which are not obvious but encoded in conversational practices, embedded in doctors' informal solidarities, invisible or impenetrable to the individual patient (e.g. Strong, 1979). Anthropologists have tended to examine a wider range of healing practices and consequently a wider range of healer–client relationships and have been particularly concerned with the extent to which healers and their clients share a diagnostic language, an 'explanatory model' of health and illness. Their interest has largely centred on the way in which the degree of cultural community or discontinuity between the healer and the sufferer may help or hinder therapeutic communication (e.g. Kleinman, 1980: 104ff).

Both medical sociologists and anthropologists have also realized that much healing activity takes place outside professional relationships altogether. There is self-medication and the healing accomplished through kin groups and in the household. There are also the folk healers, individuals who have no formal training but who claim some special knowledge or mission to heal (many spiritual healers in this country would fall into this category). However, the chapters in this volume focus on various aspects of our relationships with professional healers, looking in particular at the issue of therapeutic responsibility. What kind of commitment does the healer undertake when a patient is taken on and what is demanded of the patient? Can therapeutic responsibility be shared with other healers? If so, how does this affect the healer–patient relationship? How do institutional arrangements affect the relationship, especially where the healer is responsible not only to the patient but also to the state, to administrative or medical superiors? Should the healing bond be seen as a contractual relationship or a pastoral one?

We wanted to include not only the perspective of the social scientist but also the perspective of professionals concerned with healing – four of the chapters in the volume are written by people who are professional healers and a fifth is by a lawyer specializing in cases of medical negligence. Two of the healers are doctors and one is an alternative practitioner. The fourth is a psychoanalyst. (It seemed crucial to us to include the perspective of someone whose healing practice focused on mental distress, given both the prevalence of stress-related ailments and the uncertain status of the concept of mental illness in Western nosology.)

HEALING PRACTICE AND THE INSTITUTIONAL SETTING

Underlying the organization of this volume is the idea that medical sociology and social anthropology should be comparative in their approach.

Two kinds of comparison have been involved. First of all, we were aware that not all healing activity has as its objective the simple removal or alleviation of organic disease. Some healing relationships are directed to increasing the happiness or social adjustment of the patient, to facilitating (or limiting) fertility, to the management of incurable disease, to the support of the chronic sufferer, to the education of the patient, etc., and some of the chapters in this volume reflect this diversity of therapeutic aims.

Second, whilst the practical hegemony of 'orthodox' biomedicine must be acknowledged, there is no reason to take the kind of issues which arise in analysing official medicine as the basis for all our inquiries. We felt that the increasingly plural nature of health care in Britain (and most industrial countries) should be recognized. Stephen Fulder, on the basis of a study carried out in 1981, estimated that the number of consultations with an alternative practitioner per year in the United Kingdom might be between 11.7 and 15.4 million, that is, between 6.5 and 8.6 per cent of GP consultations (Fulder, 1989: 28). A more recent opinion poll found that 27 per cent of the sample said that they had used alternative medicine at some time in their life (MORI, 1989). Whilst earlier studies suggested that the clientele for alternative therapy was generally middle class and middle aged, there is every indication that a growing range of patients are seeking non-orthodox health professionals.

Medical anthropology has a good track record of paying due attention to the plural nature of most systems of health care provision, but this has not prevented anthropologists from alternatively succumbing to or straining against the 'medicalization of medical anthropology' (Singer, 1990: 181). In medical sociology there have been similar identity crises, the need to cut loose from biomedical moorings here tending to take the form of a stress on the agency of the patient, on the socially constructed nature of biomedical knowledge (Stacey, 1988: 1ff). In our view, recognizing the plural nature of health care provision in Western (as well as Third World countries) at the very outset allows us to ask more interesting questions about the nature of healing.

It is obvious, for example, that official and 'alternative' medicine[1] vary, not only in their power, knowledge-base and range of treatments but also in the social relationships in which both kinds of healing are embedded. The bond between healer and patient is not dyadic, though it may appear to be so. It is, at least in part, defined by many relationships outside the consulting room which structure the encounter between them. In this respect, alternative therapies differ in several ways from official medicine. They are less likely to be offered within the context of a bureaucratic structure, the majority of practitioners being engaged in solitary self-employment (although several of the chapters in this book show how a formal structure is building up within various alternative therapies). In Britain official medicine is still funded by the state and is largely free to the user at the point of delivery, whereas most alternative therapy exists outside the system of state funding (though this may change as therapies like aromatherapy and acupuncture are increasingly incorporated into NHS hospital care and fund-holding GPs begin to bring in the services of complementary therapists). Consequently the patient must pay for treatment, but independent healers are not forced to ration or be rationed in what they offer of it by budgetary constraints.

We should expect that alternative medicine, being sold on the market, would be more prone to what Freidson calls 'client control'. Where independent practitioners sell their services to individual self-selected patients, healers will be more sensitive to the lay evaluation of potential customers

than healers who practise as part of a tightly organized professional con-
fraternity, where patients frequently reach the healer by referral from
colleagues or agencies (Freidson, 1960). A look at developments in non-
orthodox medicine in the long term (see chapters in this volume by Roy
Porter and Mary Douglas) does suggest that this sensitivity to lay conceptions of good healing practice is present, though no system of healing can
afford to ignore popular conceptions of what makes for good or ill health
altogether.

However, the boundaries between official and alternative medicine are
not fixed. Many orthodox practitioners are prepared to accept alternative
medicine on the pragmatic basis that whether or not it is efficacious, if the
alternative therapist is supportive the patients find this helpful and it cannot
do any harm. And of course some orthodox practitioners have been trained
in and practise an alternative therapy themselves (mainly hypnotherapy,
homoeopathy and acupuncture). Official medicine tends to colonize
'fringe' areas of medicine once they are popular and successful. The most
recent BMA report on complementary medicine (BMA, 1993) makes it
clear that it is the growing number of patients who are resorting to alternative therapies which is causing the medical profession to consider them
seriously.[2] This document argues that since in Britain there is no statutory
restriction on the kind of therapies that may be practised and because (in
the BMA's construction of the situation) the overall responsibility for
treatment should lie in the hands of a medical practitioner, the medical
profession has a legitimate interest in ensuring that alternative practitioners
are properly trained and registered by their own professional bodies in
order that doctors may feel that they can cooperate with them and refer
patients to them. (The same arguments were used in the 1920s to the BMA
Committee of Inquiry into Psychoanalysis, see Susan Budd in this volume).

The difference between healing services which are bought and sold in
the market-place and those which are supplied through a state bureaucracy,
however disguised, has a powerfully determining effect on the patient–
healer relationship. Most of the chapters which follow refer to this. We had
not realized initially how important these aspects of the mode of delivery
would turn out to be.

There is, of course, a market for official medicine in Britain which has
produced a small private sector, and recent changes in the way in which the
National Health Service is funded have had as part of their aim to introduce
a more market-like element into the allocation and use of health care. But
there have been few attempts beyond the anecdotal to study how the
relationship between patient and doctor is affected by whether the patient
is private or not (though the subject has been more consistently studied in
the United States). One of the few exceptions (Silverman, 1987) studied the

same consultant at work in both an NHS oncology clinic and his private practice, and found the kind of superficial differences we might expect. The private practice was conducted so as to preserve the privacy and individuality of patients to a much greater degree: they were referred more rapidly to other specialists and their reactions and feelings were taken more explicitly into account. Medically their treatment was much the same. While the consultant was prepared to defer to his private patients socially and allowed them to express preferences in terms of how they were referred to, his medical authority was unchallenged. Neither he nor his patents wished to alter the assumption that he was in charge of their disease. A recent study of private patients suggests that the main reasons for choosing private orthodox medicine are 'social' rather than 'clinical' – greater privacy and dignity, sometimes also greater control over timing of appointments and treatments, a more equal relationship with the consultant (Wiles, 1993). There is little evidence of client control over the purely clinical aspects of private orthodox practice, probably because of the strong institutional connections between private and public purveyors of orthodox medicine (most private consultants also practise within the NHS), and a high degree of professional unity and common culture among orthodox doctors regardless of which sector they practise in.

A further 'institutional' factor is the legal framework within which health care systems operate, which influences their structure and use (not totally: in the Netherlands and some other European countries the practice of complementary medicine by persons other than medically qualified doctors is forbidden by law, but the state has effectively anticipated the liberalization of the official position, and non-medical practitioners are seldom prosecuted (BMA, 1993: 18)). Two of the chapters in this book (by Margaret Stacey and Robert Sumerling) discuss (and disagree over) issues related to the regulation of orthodox medical practitioners. Margaret Stacey argues that the present system of self-regulation adopted by the medical profession does not work well enough for it to be recommended for the complementary therapies. Robert Sumerling points out that healer–practitioner relationships are in fact governed by the law but that if there is widespread resort to suing practitioners for malpractice, patients may be protected but insurance premiums will rise enormously and both orthodox and alternative treatments will become considerably more expensive. Another possible effect of the perceived 'malpractice crisis' is that doctors may respond simply by trying to improve relationships with patients through better communication (they are then thought less likely to complain) without necessarily addressing the question of technical competence (Annandale, 1989).

CONSTRUCTIONS OF THE 'PATIENT'

Many orthodox anxieties about alternative medicine are similar to those about private medicine. They are often expressed in terms of the possibility that practitioners may take advantage of vulnerable patients, distressed and socially weakened by their illnesses, to secure their compliance for treatments which are never going to cure them, thereby failing to obtain an orthodox treatment which would offer some hope of improvement. In fact there is much ambiguity in current discourse about medicine as to whether patients should be constructed as persons who are potentially in a morally vulnerable state because of their illness and who must therefore be protected by a responsible profession, or as self-responsible consumers whose illness must not be regarded as in itself denying their capacity to make choices in accordance with their own priorities and the information which responsible professionals should offer them.

It is certainly difficult to act as autonomous beings when we are very ill – we may be more anxious, more passive and in need of more support and reassurance than when we are well. Can we be expected to make appropriate choices when racked with pain? The notion of consent to treatment assumes that we must be treated as though we can. But doctors do not always find the consequences of such an approach easy to live with, especially where the patient or his/her proxy questions or even refuses treatment which the doctor regards as life-saving (see Alderson, 1990).

This ambiguity is referred to in the British Medical Association's document *Philosophy and Practice of Medical Ethics*:

> In the past the doctor/patient relationship tended to rely heavily upon a paternalistic approach by the doctor. Originally this approach arose because of the inequality of knowledge between them. . . . This attitude cannot continue in the face of developments in general education and the advent of the modern media of mass communication. Increasingly patients have begun expressing a desire to know what is wrong with them and to understand the action taken by doctors. . . . Simultaneously, more emphasis is being placed on the patients assuming responsibility for their own health, especially concerning the effects of their own way of life on their health.
>
> (BMA, 1988: 7–8)

Leaving aside the question of whether the orthodox medical profession's construction of its own past is historically accurate, is this model of the self-responsible consumer/patient what sick people actually want? Certainly it is widely held (see Taylor, 1984; also Mary Douglas's chapter in this volume) that the increasing popularity of alternative therapies has to do with dissatisfaction with a system of medicine that tends to treat the body as a machine to be mended rather than as one aspect of a person who is also a social and spiritual being. On the other hand a recent study in Australia suggested that laypeople desired a GP in whom they could put trust, and showed few signs of preferring a more egalitarian model or wanting more control over treatment (Lupton *et al.*, 1991). Probably much depends on how we ask the question and which kind of patients we have in mind. There is no reason to suppose that laypeople agree on the kind of healer–patient relationship that suits them any more than they will agree on, say, the kind of education they want for their children.

Most patients of alternative therapy and also many patients of psycho-therapists and infertility clinics, psychosexual medicine, etc. will fall into the 'chronic' category. Several chapters in this volume deal with such forms of healing in which not only do therapeutic objectives consist of more than simply 'curing' a defined and understood 'disease' or 'condition', but also sufferers themselves are likely to come to the encounter already potentially more anxious as to whether they will get what they hope for from the treatment, possibly also more knowledgeable about their problem from long familiarity with it. The chapters by Susan Budd and Gillian Vanhegan suggest that possibly both the 'self-responsible consumer' and the 'trusting in professional wisdom' construction of the patient may be irrelevant simply because they are too static: where the healing encounter is conceived as a personal *process* (whether of self-understanding, coming to terms with one's condition, arriving at appro-priate decisions, etc.) the patients themselves, and not just their bodies, are transformed.

One of the issues we have had to come to terms with in the course of editing this volume is the diversity of professional constructions of the 'patient'. Orthodox medical practice constructs the patient as *inexpert* in relation to the physician's technical and scientific expertise. Some forms of alternative medicine reject this construction in favour of emphasis on the *singularity* of the individual patient, whose problems will be untangled by the joint efforts of the professional and the patient in a process of discovery, a journey towards self-understanding for the patient (see Ursula Sharma's chapter in this volume).

Social scientists have their own constructions of the patient. In medical sociology there has been much stress on the *agency* of the patient, an emphasis on the capacity of patients to use their own knowledge, to decide not to consult medical professionals, or to resist the power they hold. Anthropologists have tended to construct the patient in terms of *rationality*, perhaps to rescue the 'other' from the charge of impenetrable irrationality, stressing the logic of the patient's illness behaviour, even if it is logical only within a set of cultural notions about disease and illness which the researcher does not share (see Young, 1981). Both these social scientific constructions of the patient play down the emotional dimensions of illness, which are, of course, what the therapist usually has to confront.

However, these are all constructions of the patient by professionals of one kind or another. The question of how patients construct *themselves* is unanswerable in general terms because in the world outside the consulting room the category of patient dissolves. In that world sick people are not patients, but persons who may or may not construct their identity in terms of the illness they have or in terms of their use of a particular kind of treatment. 'Patients' may form self-help groups (often encouraged by orthodox medicine) or support groups for a particular kind of healing (homoeopathy has generated users' pressure groups since the nineteenth century and recently chiropractic patients have formed an association). But many people seek ways of acknowledging illness without accepting a 'patient role'. Thus among AIDS activists there has been a shift from the passivity implied by the term 'AIDS victim' to the notion of a 'person with AIDS', and, more recently, 'persons living with AIDS' (Pollak *et al.*, 1992: 102). It is a practical problem for therapists of all kinds that in a complex, multicultural (postmodern?) society they cannot know in advance of meeting a patient how that person will wish to construct his or her own role in relation to the professional healer and the process of treatment. Some people may resort to alternative medicine in protest against orthodox medicine's construction of the patient role (see Taylor, 1984; also Mary Douglas's chapter in this volume); others may be seen by both orthodox and alternative practitioners as far too passive in relation to both their illness and the healer, too inclined to assume that they can hand over responsibility to someone who will cure them without any work or understanding on their part.

INTERPROFESSIONAL COOPERATION AND THERAPEUTIC RESPONSIBILITY

Where sick people opt for treatments outside the scope and organization of orthodox medicine, how far can doctors continue to exercise the total therapeutic responsibility which their own ethics and professional traditions favour?

> It is good medical practice in the UK for one doctor to be responsible for the overall management of a patient's illness. This system helps to ensure that a patient with a particular complaint is assessed as a whole.
> (BMA, 1988: 10)

This theory of the doctor–patient relationship with its assumption of the over-riding competence of doctors to know what is good for patients is no doubt behind the General Medical Council ruling that doctors may refer patients to alternative therapists provided that they maintain overall therapeutic responsibility. It is a matter of current debate among complementary therapists' professional bodies as to whether they should accept this construction of the relationship between orthodox and non-orthodox medicine, some conceding the orthodox doctor's right to diagnose whilst others claim that if their own skills and knowledge have any validity at all then they should be free to accept full therapeutic responsibility for their patients. It is not clear to us whether this would make very much difference to the legal situation of therapist and patient in the event of a case of negligence being brought against the therapist. But at a time when the public construction of the patient (vulnerable and dependent or consumerist and self-responsible?) is very much open to revision (and also the public construction of the alternative therapist – commercial quacks or responsible professionals?) it might make the world of moral difference.

The recent growth of alternative therapies of various kinds is generally attributed to the increasing pressures of time and medical specialization inside a health service which is overwhelmed by its very success in mobilizing popular demand. Studies of the resort to alternative therapies suggest that the majority of users do not reject orthodox medicine and 'believe in' an alternative set of medical ideas; rather they find that the treatment they receive for a particular complaint does not seem to be satisfactory and they turn to an alternative therapy in the hope of finding a cure or a better way of managing it. Once there, they may find that the chosen therapy has a rather different view on the nature and genesis of illness. As Richenda Power's chapter in this volume shows, a responsible alternative practitioner will usually need to discuss with the patient the implications of differences in approach between orthodox medicine and his or her own discipline. Patients may embrace this new view enthusiastically and refer themselves to alternative therapy for other complaints, or they may continue to see alternative therapy as having a limited and complementary role (Sharma, 1992). Olivier Faure's (1992) analysis of the clientele of a well known Parisian homoeopath during the inter-war period suggests that this division of users of alternative therapy into the convinced/committed and the experimental/transient is by no means a new phenomenon. The 'transient' patients may also find alternative medicine ineffective. Such patients are understandably unpopular with both kinds of healer, who are each likely to feel that the other side condemns their type of treatment for failing to cure the incurable.

Alternative therapies are not a homogeneous group. They differ widely in respect of knowledge-base and with regard to the way they see their relationship with orthodox medicine. Within each therapy practitioners may vary – some would like to cooperate with orthodox doctors, others may feel that they are engaged in a different enterprise altogether. Consequently they cannot be assumed to be enamoured of each other. Doctors also differentiate between alternative therapies in their own attitudes. More doctors are likely to recommend osteopaths and counsellors for instance than would recommend radionics or iridology. Doctors may see particular therapies as having knowledge-bases compatible with orthodox medicine and as offering a relatively limited pragmatic form of help. The alternative practitioner may not agree, but some will decide that it is not politic to stress their rather different underlying approach. David Peters's chapter in this volume explores the practical difficulties of trying to integrate orthodox and different kinds of alternative medicine in the same healing centre, which raises all the issues of inter-professional collaboration that have already been recorded in relation to cooperation between doctors and other professionals within the NHS, especially nurses and midwives (see Calliope Farsides's chapter). Some alternative therapies are unlikely to welcome doctors who have received brief training in their specialisms and then proceed to practise them, but here they run into the complex issues to do with the relative power of different kinds of therapy and the way in which state support for official medicine affects relations between conventional and alternative practitioners (issues explored by Richenda Power, Margaret Stacey, Roy Porter and Susan Budd in this volume).

It is often possible for someone trained in orthodox medicine to make sense of another discipline's healing modalities where there is the will to do so. Sudhir Kakar (1982), an Indian trained in Western psychiatry, has recorded his sympathetic attempts to understand Indian healing practices as applied to mental distress. This process is something like that of the anthropologist who struggles to understand and translate the categories of another culture without reducing them simply to categories in his or her own. Thus Krause (1989) describes the Punjabi concept of 'sinking heart' and compares it with Western categories like heart disease, depression, 'Type A personality'. She shows that whilst these categories are not translatable into one another, the systems are mutually intelligible. Yet Richenda Power's chapter suggests that the relationship between healing modes remains asymmetrical in many ways; responsible alternative practitioners need to know much more about current orthodox treatments for the conditions their patients present than orthodox practitioners are ever likely to be expected to know about alternative treatments for the same conditions.

On the other hand, orthodox medicine itself is also heterogeneous. Doctors in some specialisms may privately consider others – psychiatrists for instance – as little better than quacks. Some, as Mary Douglas points out, actually practise as holistically within the constraints of the NHS as some non-orthodox counterparts. But their situation and professional relations are more closely regulated by the state and, as Margaret Stacey shows, by a lengthy process of common socialization which trains doctors not to criticize each other to patients. It is widely assumed, perhaps less so recently, that doctors are more trustworthy and responsible individuals than alternative practitioners. Certainly doctors who are publicly disgraced usually attract comment about their special position of trust. It can be argued that the lengthy training doctors receive does make them feel more confident and supported in tackling such responsibilities than those complementary practitioners who have very short periods of professional training, and that the integration of doctors within complex institutions may provide them with more support in dealing with the pressures which needy patients can put upon them than those complementary practitioners who work in isolation. The issue of sexual relations between healers and patients has been much discussed recently (Rutter, 1989) and is touched upon by Margaret Stacey, Robert Sumerling, Susan Budd and Gillian Vanhegan in this volume.

MEDICAL RESPONSIBILITIES IN THE MODERN WORLD

The nature of healing may largely be determined by the epidemiology of a given society. Many of the problems which people bring to doctors in industrialized societies are not of the acute type for which orthodox treatment is likely to be effective and rapid. Our attitude to our broken leg, or, for that matter, to the doctor who treats it, will not interfere much with the healing process and the doctor can afford to ignore it.[3] But if we develop diabetes, asthma or multiple sclerosis, our relation to our ailment may be lifelong and how we live with it and manage these conditions is very much up to our own efforts. Our relationship with the doctor may become more problematic, especially where there is uncertainty of prognosis or outcome of treatment. In a study of patient–practitioner relationships, Calnan points out that people who consult for transient ailments may well express satisfaction with a directive doctor; if they do not like the diagnosis or the treatment they have no need to challenge it. They comply or not, as they think fit, and the illness will clear up in the end anyway. In the case of chronic disease, patients see more of the doctor, but also are liable to become more 'expert' in their own diseases and hence more likely to express criticisms of the doctor's view (Calnan, 1984: 83). In chronic illness we may become frustrated because the doctor cannot rid us of these conditions in the way we would like and may find it hard to acknowledge our feelings about our defective body. Doctors in turn may become frustrated by the social and psychological circumstances which may prevent chronic patients from living in what they regard as an optimal way. Under such circumstances some patients will turn to alternative medicine and other forms of healing.

Modern biomedicine is responsible for major developments in the control of infectious disease and has made dramatic progress in areas such as in utero surgery. These relatively recent advances mean that many of the problems which modern doctors must deal with are those deriving from the processes of age and degeneration as life expectancy is extended. These conditions can seldom be reversed, though they may be alleviated. Effective medicine in the sense of medicine which produces the steady and conclusive relief of symptoms involves relatively limited contact with doctors and if we see more of them we are likely to be chronically ill.

At the same time, expectations have risen enormously. We expect to be well in old age in a way that previous generations did not. Wellness is 'normal' in an almost moral sense; smoking or obesity may be even regarded as disqualification to employment and the role of chronic invalid is scarcely regarded as legitimate. Doctors must be more concerned with prevention (health education, immunization). The medicalization of many conditions not previously regarded as under the control of medicine has expanded doctors' responsibilities to the infertile, the pregnant and parturient, the mentally disturbed and the anxious, involving doctors in many activities where the outcome is broader than simply the cure of symptoms, the removal of disease. The responsibilities of the doctor are no longer clear-cut and, here again, patient discontent may surface where there is disagreement about what the object of medical activity is held to be. Is the responsibility of the obstetrician, for instance, simply to deliver a healthy baby with minimum risk to the mother, or to deploy every known kind of prenatal test to ensure a 'perfect' baby at all costs? If it is a characteristic of modern Western societies, as some have suggested, to see the allocation of human responsibility for misfortune as very important, then the healing professions are bound to attract some of that blame, and it is reasonable for them to ask whether they may not be better protected were there societal agreements about limits to what the patient is entitled to expect from therapeutic interventions of any kind (see Mary Douglas's chapter in this volume).

This brings us to an area which many people feel so painful as to be taboo. If resources are limited, as they always must be, how can doctors reconcile their responsibility to do what they can for each patient with the inevitable need to ration the time and help they can give? There can be no doubt that doctors are often forced through pressure of time to behave in an authoritarian way, substituting prescriptions for attentive listening to the patient's view of the situation. The trouble is that this deprives the doctors of one of the most important medicines they have to give: the healing bond itself. Gillian Vanhegan discusses how in an area like psychosexual medicine the skilful and compassionate doctor must nimbly move between behaving in a relatively 'scientific' way, in which she must consider the patient's physical problems as an objective problem and swiftly identify medical or surgical remedies, and being responsive to the patient's emotional demands, which often require that she does not respond to the demand for immediate treatment but encourages patients to explore their own dilemmas. These two relationships require that the doctor fit into two different kinds of 'transference' relationship; in effect be two different kinds of people. The conditions in which the second kind of medicine can be given require more relief from pressure, both external and within the mind of the doctor and patient, than the first.[4]

Many doctors are uncomfortable with the idea that the relationships that they form with their patients can be crucial to the patients' satisfaction or otherwise with their treatment. It denies the positivist assumption that sharp divisions can be made between mind and body and brain. Having been taught to mistrust the placebo effect as though it were at worst a kind of cheating, at best something which (in clinical trials) they must aim to improve upon if the treatment under consideration is to be regarded as worthwhile, it is difficult for doctors to accept that it can offer the most potent power to cure, although the statistics themselves repeatedly suggest its importance. At the other end many social scientists tend to assume an extreme cultural relativism which states that illness and cure is simply what each person or culture says it is. This may be a permissible stance for the purposes of social science research but is it an appropriate position for those who, say, are responsible for the allocation of public resources or for the preparation of legislation to regulate healing professions? Our own view is that the process of healing has many components, and whilst we think that what we have called the healing bond is a crucial component of the process, we do not suggest that effective healing practice is *only* a matter of good relationships with patients, thereby denying the role of technical interventions, whatever these may be for a given mode of healing (surgical procedures, the prescription of medicines, the manipulation of bodies or even manipulation of symbols) which may be performed competently or incompetently.

But this does not dispose of the problem of what constitutes a cure. Who is to decide on efficacy? The healer, the patient or some alliance of the two? There is considerable debate at present about the demonstration of efficacy in alternative therapy. Orthodox doctors have conventionally held that only clinical trials which satisfy their own scientific criteria of proof will do. Some alternative therapists question whether it is the business of orthodox doctors to stand in judgement over therapies which may involve quite different notions of the nature of health and healing from those of bio-medicine. Arguably, both sides overlook the judgement of the patients and the criteria which they might wish to use. Clearly other bodies are involved in this – the law, for instance, where, as Robert Summerling points out, issues of whether the patient did or did not receive reasonable care or was even abused tend to end up. Within some systems of traditional medicine, the individual is often treated in the context of the community. Illness or misfortune are often seem as a symptom that relationships between the individual and the local community have gone wrong and need to be re-examined.

Those who have studied healing in non-European cultures have frequently remarked that some kinds of healing do not call upon the involvement of the sick person alone, but of his or her kin for instance, or of a cult group (see Janzen, 1978; Turner, 1967). In some cases the rituals or therapeutic activities may be undertaken by others while the patient remains passive (Skultans, 1987). Possibly the Western therapeutic tradition is unusual in holding to a model of healer–patient relationship which is regarded as (ideally at any rate) a confidential relationship between two *individuals*. The attempts of the government to return the care of the long-term mentally ill back to the responsibility of the 'community', how-ever motivated, go counter to a therapeutic tradition of possessive individu-alism. (What has been said here of orthodox medicine is largely true also of the alternative therapies as they are practised in Britain and most Western countries: some therapists may say that they would *like* to treat the patient's family but in practice it is individuals who present themselves for treatment. Often, from the point of view of the therapists, the wrong individual comes.)

THE PATIENT'S ROLE IN HEALING

Ultimately there is something rather enigmatic about what actually heals us. Perhaps an example would make things more vivid. In 1986 the travel writer Alexander Frater (1991) woke one morning to find that he had no feeling in his feet. The condition progressed and he rationalized it – a virus picked up in the East, or a psychosomatic phenomenon. When it worsened he consulted his GP, who agreed that it was serious and referred him to the National Hospital for Nervous Diseases. The doctors here were equally non-plussed. The elaboration and sophistication of the diagnostic tests were impressive, but served mainly to disprove possibilities. Finally he was diagnosed as suffering from a congenital defect at the top of the spine which had been aggravated by travelling over rough roads in China. The symptoms 'might or might not go away of their own accord. There was no known medical treatment'. Frater's half-hearted attempts to convey his distress and anxiety to his various doctors were side-stepped. The doctors did not evade him altogether but pointed out that there was nothing medicine could do for him. He was discharged with a warning to avoid jarring his neck and slid into a depression and invalidism and consumed rather too much whisky. Several months later he had a chance meeting in the outpatients' clinic with an energizing Indian couple who reminded him of a long forgotten project to travel northwards with the Indian monsoon. He went to see his neurologist, who commented that he looked cheerful and asked after the neck. 'I can live with it', he said for the first time, and made plans to visit India.

Arriving in Kerala he found that in India medicine was less clearly demarcated from other activities. He visited a healer, Mr Nair, who had inherited his position as head of a clinic and martial arts school and would hand it on in turn to his son. Mr Nair immediately recognized that there was something wrong with Frater's neck and that it was something to do with a traffic accident suffered in the past, but, like the Western neurologist, could offer no cure. He could not mend him, but he could treat his general health and spirits with a combination of massage and oils at the beginning of the monsoon, 'when body and mind heal best'. Frater did not go into treatment with him, but he did get better, or at least his symptoms disappear from the narrative.

This enigmatic tale can stand for many stories that we read and, as practitioners, are told about patients' searches for healing and health. The two sorts of medicine were agreed on diagnosis, and that they could do nothing for the neck itself. But whereas 'high-tech' Western medicine confined it to the symptoms and their possible causes, Mr Nair was more concerned with Frater's general health and spirits. Neither aspired to cure the neck – so what did? Was the condition self-limiting and would it have gone away in any case? Did the energizing effect of the Indian couple in the outpatients' clinic remind him of reasons for living and give him the confidence to try, i.e. they effected an instant transference cure? Or did the lifting of depression have a physical effect on his body, enabling it to heal? Did he simply decide to stop living as an invalid, the solution he himself seems to accept? Was it indeed the monsoon and the excitement and overflowing energy that it released which made the difference? Western medicine's diagnostic tests had relieved him of the fear of multiple sclerosis; often a condition is much more tolerable when we know what has caused it, and to be told that we definitely do not have a more serious disease can be enormously important.

To tellers of these stories it really does not matter; when the pain goes, when the cure seems to be found, that is the end of the affair. But just because of this it is often difficult to assess or compare the results of different therapies. As the patient moves between different practitioners, each is given a slightly different snapshot of the ailment and each adds his or her own perspective to the map in the patient's mind.

It is because of this that a popular literature has sprung up around the healing encounter which tends to stress the dramatic effects that any new kind of intervention can have. This literature tells us how the doctor, or more commonly the alternative healer, sees someone for whom previous remedies have not worked and offers his or her new perspective on treatment. The patient embraces it with enthusiasm, and may continue to be treated and to be appreciative, or may cease to attend, saying that he or she has recovered. The healer's view of the efficacy of his or her treatment is reinforced and the patient is unlikely to complain. But because such accounts concentrate on successful cases, we cannot make accurate overall maps of illness and treatment from them, therefore we cannot follow what happens when the patient is not satisfied with the treatment and drifts away. Much that is relevant to the patient's experience of illness does not take place in the consulting room at all and may not even be known to the healer who is currently treating the patient. It is likely that some chronic patients move along trajectories trying many therapies, often abandoning regimes they find difficult or uncongenial. They will fail to turn up to appointments but will not confront the healer with their dissatisfactions regarding either the social or clinical aspects of the treatment. Therapists know that other patients keep turning up at the same practitioner, becoming 'difficult' or 'fat envelope' patients for whom, it is tacitly agreed, nothing is really going to work. At any point they may decide that what they have is incurable but can be lived with, and at any point some conditions simply get better.

It is only those practitioners who either see the same patient over a very long period of time, or those (such as psychotherapists) who encourage patients to talk about their negative and hopeless feelings about their treatment, who are likely to be in touch with what happens when the healing bond fails. Social scientists have little to say about therapeutic failure except in broad terms. They do not claim competence to judge issues relating to the efficacy of the treatment and when they have studied the social dimensions of the healer–patient interaction it has generally been in general institutional terms. They seldom have the opportunity to observe how either patients or healers behave in cases of therapeutic failure or where communication between them breaks down. Furthermore, it is difficult to conduct research which looks at people who are not currently in treatment or who move between different kinds of healer, because they are harder to identify and stay with. From the point of view of the practitioner, however, the distinction between healer–patient relationships where the treatment works and those where it does not is crucial.

The healing bond rests on the assumption that the healer has something to offer which can make a difference. Healers are not passive: they will have a view about the condition, as to whether it can be cured or whether the patients can only be supported in coming to terms with it, how far the patient should be expected or encouraged to re-arrange his or her life to cope with or end the disability, and so on. But issues of who is to blame never lie far below the surface. The more emphasis that has been placed on the moral or emotional aspects of the healing bond, the more both parties will feel angry, let down, recriminatory or guilty when it does not appear to have worked. In this volume we look at the healing process mainly from the point of view of what is transacted between healer and patient in the clinic or consulting room, but we must remember that sick people may or may not work towards their own cure, and that we must all come to terms with the limitations of the healing art itself.

NOTES

1 It will be noted that in the chapter which follows we use a variety of terms to define different kinds of healing. When we use the term 'doctor' we mean someone who practises conventional biomedicine. The term 'healer' refers to a practitioner of any form of healing, conventional or 'alternative'. We have not attempted any further standardization of terms for orthodox/conventional/ official medicine and non-orthodox/alternative/complementary therapies because we believe these diverse terminologies point to a real confusion in the world about how to define each group and what relations should be between them (though individual contributors have used terms which conform with their personal views of such relationships).

   Similarly what do we call the people who use the healing services of such professionals? Some social scientists have objected to the term 'patient' since it implies a passive relationship with a healer rather than active health-seeking and obscures the efforts which people make to heal themselves. And should we use the same term for those who consult alternative and orthodox healers? Some would prefer the term 'patient' to be reserved for someone who uses orthodox medicine. But 'client' and 'customer' carry overtones which may be appropriate in some contexts and not others. We have tended to use 'patient' to refer to people who use the services of healers of any kind, since this book is mainly about what happens between the sick person and the professional practitioner rather than about the sick role in general.

2 Readers should note that most of the chapters in this volume were written before the publication of the 1993 BMA report on complementary medicine, which only appeared as we were in the final stages of the editing process.

3 This is not always so. See Sacks (1986) for a fascinating account by a neurologist who broke his leg – it was healed, but he could not move it until his emotional attitude had changed.

4   We are talking about orthodox medicine here but in our view it is likely that this alternation between clinical detachment and engagement with the patient's subjectivity is characteristic of most healing traditions.

REFERENCES

Alderson, P. (1990) *Choosing for Children*, Oxford: Oxford University Press.

Annandale, E.C. (1989) 'The Malpractice Crisis and the Doctor–Patient Relationship', *Sociology of Health and Illness*, 11(1): 1–23.

BMA (1988) *Philosophy and Practice of Medical Ethics*, London: BMA.

BMA (1993) *Complementary Medicine: New Approaches to Good Practice*, Oxford: Oxford University Press.

Calnan, M. (1984) 'Clinical Uncertainty: is it a Problem for the Doctor–Patient Relationship?', *Sociology of Health and Illness*, 6(1): 74–85.

Faure, O. (1992) *Praticiens, Patients et Militants de l'Homéopathie (1800–1940)*, Lyons: Boiron.

Frater, A. (1991) *Chasing the Monsoon*, New York: Viking.

Freidson, E. (1960) 'Client Control and Medical Practice', *American Journal of Sociology*, 65: 374–82.

Fulder, S. (1989) *Handbook of Complementary Medicine* (rev. and updated edn), Sevenoaks: Coronet Books.

Janzen, J. (1978) *The Quest for Therapy in Lower Zaïre*, Berkeley: University of California Press.

Kakar, S. (1982) *Shamans, Mystics and Doctors: A Psychological Enquiry into India and its Healing Traditions*, New York: Alfred A. Knopf.

Kleinman, A. (1980) *Patients and Healers in the Context of Culture*, Berkeley: University of California Press.

Krause, I.-B. (1989) 'Sinking Heart: A Punjabi Communication of Distress', *Social Science and Medicine*, 29(4): 563–75.

Lupton, D., Donaldson, C. and Lloyd, P. (1991) 'Caveat Emptor or Blissful Ignorance? Patients and the Consumerist Ethos', *Social Science and Medicine*, 33(5): 559–68.

MORI (Market and Opinion Research International) (1989) *Alternative Medicine* (research conducted for *The Times* newspaper).

Pollak, M., Paicheler, G. and Pierret, J. (1992) *AIDS: A Problem for Sociological Research*, London: Sage.

Rutter, P. (1989) *Sex in the Forbidden Zone*, London: Mandala.

Sacks, O. (1986) *A Leg to Stand On*, London: Pan.

Sharma, U. (1992) *Complementary Medicine Today: Practitioners and Patients*, London and New York: Tavistock/Routledge.

Silverman, D. (1987) *Communications and Medical Practice. Social Relations in the Clinic*, London: Sage.

Singer, M. (1990) 'Reinventing Medical Anthropology: Toward a Critical Realignment', *Social Science and Medicine*, 30(2): 179–87.

Skultans, V. (1987) 'Trance and the Management of Mental Illness', *Anthropology Today*, 3(1): 2–4.

Stacey, M. (1988) *The Sociology of Health and Healing: A Textbook*, London: Unwin Hyman (reprinted 1991, London: Routledge).

Strong, P. (1979) *The Ceremonial Order of the Clinic. Patients, Doctors and Medical Bureaucrats*, London: Routledge & Kegan Paul.

Taylor, C.R. (1984) 'Alternative Medicine and the Medical Encounter in Britain and the United States', in J. Warren Salmon (ed.), *Alternative Medicines: Popular and Policy Perspectives*, London: Tavistock.

Turner, V. (1967) *The Forest of Symbols*, Ithaca, NY, and London: Cornell University Press.

Wiles, R. (1993) 'Women and Private Medicine', *Sociology of Health and Illness*, 15(1): 68–85.

Young, A. (1981) 'When Rational Men Fall Ill', *Culture, Medicine and Psychiatry*, 5: 317–35.

Part I
General perspectives

1 The construction of the physician

A cultural approach to medical fashions

Mary Douglas

THE SOCIAL CONSTRUCTION OF THE PHYSICIAN

Some friends explain their preference for complementary medicine by saying either that it is 'holistic' or that it respects spiritual values, or both. Here I propose to put this preference in the context of a widespread leaning towards what I will call 'gentleness'. There have always been some people concerned for animal welfare, but now that concern is widespread. There have always been vegetarians, but good restaurants did not always offer a vegetarian menu, as they now are obliged to do if they want to stay in business. New religions depict a compassionate image of God. In a quasi-religious mood, environmentalists try to make us sensitive to nature's needs. Alternative medicine invokes tender sensibilities on behalf of the body. There has always been alternative or complementary medicine but now the sheer numbers of patients are impressive, and increasing (Sermeus, 1987). Animals, religion, ecology and medicine, there is a case for studying them together under a single rubric, the option for gentleness.

A word about the term 'gentleness' is in order. Of course it is relative. Some forms of complementary medicine are pretty brutal, like chiropractic; some traditional medication is painless. But surely we can agree that cutting up flesh and bone or drawing blood are violent therapies compared with remedies coming in the form of perfumes and oils, and that manipulation is less intrusive than the surgeon's knife. Acupuncture involves needle pricks sited away from the painful region, which do not hurt or even draw blood. Laying on of hands relieves pain without so much as touching the sufferer's skin. These are the new style of therapy, light oils from flowers and seeds to pamper the tired muscles, hypnotic trance to unknot deep worry, infusions of herbs to invigorate the spirit. As to diagnosis, it does no violence to the patient's bodily privacy. Because the state of the whole is manifest in its parts, the patient does not even need to undress. The global condition can be assessed through the eye, or the foot.

Though there is the possibility that the therapist, too, is kinder and more sympathetic, this will not do for an explanation of the preference. Much more relevant is the kind of theories that the therapist will invoke: global, holistic, spiritual, rather than local, partial and physical. Here I am particularly interested in the construction of the therapist as a guide to a different reality. The argument will be that two polarized types of therapy contain in their mutually opposed imagery two types of therapist. If we are interested in the bond between patient and doctor we must be interested in the way these constructions are made.

In 'The Social Construction of the Patient' (1985) Claudine Herzlich and Janine Pierret present a perspective within which it is wrong to take disease to be a person's bodily condition alone. 'A person's experiences and his lay conceptions of sickness cannot be separated from macro-social phenomena.' I am saying the same about the healing bond. Herzlich and Pierret go on to describe how the idea of sickness has been constructed in historic times and different places, in each case as an integral part of a world-view. It should hardly be necessary to say that the healing bond is socially patterned, too, and that social patterns can and should be studied within a holistic framework.

HOLISM

Although complementary is now the preferred term, there is a sense in which the old name of 'alternative' was right insofar as this therapeutic effort caters to a different kind of demand for health care, coming from a different source, bearing a different flag. It is alternative in the full counter-cultural sense, 'spiritual' in contrast to 'material'. Consequently strictly medical comparisons afford too narrow a basis for interpreting the key word, 'holism'. Present-day medical holism is a philosophy of the body which does not grow out of the history of Western medicine. Otherwise you might say that our family doctor takes a holistic view of medicine. The smallest ailment, and she is ready to think ahead to its furthest possible repercussions through the whole range of bodily parts and medical knowledge. Consult her about a swollen shin bone, and she immediately anticipates a thrombosis; go to her with earache and she warns against danger of a tumour on the brain; call about your feet and she suspects possible Parkinsonism. I personally appreciate having the diagnostic resources of Western medicine placed at my disposal. But this is not at all what is meant by medical holism. Our doctor's holism stops at the boundaries of the body and stays within the boundaries of the medical profession, whereas holistic medicine takes global account of the patient's whole personality and spiritual environment.

Western medicine over its history has gradually separated itself from spiritual matters. In a pluralist democracy the varied religious beliefs of the population must be respected. It would be improper for medical practitioners to foist their own religious views on their patients. Religion was split off from medicine, psychic troubles from bodily ones, then the treatment of one limb from another, flesh from bone, skin from sub-cutaneous, organs from each other, one virus distinguished from another, and diseases cross-cutting the classification by anatomic parts. As its history of research has been a process of specializing, so now the body itself is parcelled out among a host of specialists. It all comes together in a general theory of living beings, but that does not take account of the psyche. The complementary medicine that is being discussed in this volume is neither encroaching on the churches nor offering to its patients the opportunity of embracing an alternative religious cult. It draws on ancient theories of how living beings are related to the cosmos, and a set of theories about the connection between psychic and physical existence: it is, in short, a cultural alternative to Western philosophic traditions.

Personal preference is not much of an explanation when one theory about what the world is like and how bodies behave opposes another. When the same population is divided in its adherence to one or the other worldview, cultural conflict is present. As the people hear the terms of the conflict, competition between cultural principles spreads; soon no one will be able to stay neutral as to meat-eating, or religion, or concern for the environment. Even medicine may become a ground for testing allegiance.

SPIRITUAL VERSUS MATERIAL VALUES

When I ask my friends to tell me what they mean by saying that they prefer a medical tradition that is more spiritual, they answer with a series of contrasts. The idea of spirituality in medical practice is contrasted in these conversations with materiality, physicality, violence. My other friends, who use conventional therapies, rebuke me for accepting the contrast: how can modern Western medicine be more physical, materialist or violent? But the contrast is not absurd. We have just specified the relatively incorporeal treatments which earn alternative therapies the adjective of gentle.

The contrast of spiritual and material is used in a medical context to contrast with or to complement physical needs and physicalist remedies. The claim that the new therapeutic tradition is spiritual would be valid insofar as it uses a range of symbolism that goes beyond the clinic to embrace the whole person in the whole universe. In a political context, the label 'material' becomes a criticism of holders of wealth and power. What the powerful wealthy say in defence of their ways is likely to be judged materialist; the other label, 'spiritual', is appropriated by the cultural critics for their own preferences: by the logic of opposition spiritual is incompatible with accumulating power or wealth. A preacher who makes a fortune tends to be suspected of materialist objectives.

There are many other contexts in which objects and conduct are ranked on a scale from material to spiritual. Gross/subtle, vulgar/refined, rough/ smooth, harsh/gentle, brutal/tender, mechanical/personal, divine/human, pure/impure, are universal forms of evaluation. Between science and the humanities we use the scale of hard/soft. Tension between material and spiritual values is always present. What I am calling the option for gentleness is a surfacing of a new trend, against the material, against vulgar, harsh, rough, hard, brutal, mechanical and impure, complementary to a preference for spirituality.

In certain phases of human history, or in certain segments of society, the option for spirituality becomes an irresistible demand. We should make a first attempt to lay a trail that will find connections between the present option and other such movements. The rejection of animal sacrifice in early Hinduism and the still vital Hindu movement towards ritual purity and against bloodshed is a vivid example. The debate conducted between Greek philosophers in the first centuries BC against cruelty to animals, including eating or sacrificing them, is another example. By reflecting on previous movements in the same direction, contemporary cultural conflicts about the treatment of the body, the environment and the animals can be seen as a total social phenomenon.

THE CHALLENGE TO MEDICAL ANTHROPOLOGY

Any civilization which takes pride in its medicine has its own diagnostic classifications. The Lele, a people in Zaïre, class swellings of all kinds together, which means that boils and abscesses come under the same general rubric as swollen bellies and pregnancies, all caused by fertility spirits. The same people consider that pulmonary complaints are due to a tendency for ribs to get crossed and to rub against one another, causing wheezing sounds; they diagnose certain stomach pains as caused by the liver refusing to lie flat in its proper place. In the Punjab the symptoms of stress are described as a sinking of the heart (Krause, 1989). In the history of modern medicine there were stages in which the position of organs was a principal cause of disorder. Female hysteria, for example, was thought to be caused by the womb wandering away from base. But if we were consistently to try to trace differences in exotic medical theory by relating them to earlier phases in the growth of our own, the conclusion is prejudged: the other medicine, alternative to our own, is bound to be found primitive, despised and misjudged as an early stage of evolution.

Such a condescending conclusion would be entirely false, as there is no reason to think that other medical practices ever belonged to the same kind of process as early modern medicine, to say nothing of being set on the same evolutionary path. There is always the problem of finding the right diagnostic levels for comparison. When a patient tells a modern doctor that he suffers from heart burn, the doctor does not take the description for diagnosis. Some mental troubles are currently diagnosed in Western medicine as due to physical pressure on the brain; 'foreign bodies' or 'water' can mysteriously cause pain by getting into the knee. Some kind of reality is being described by patient or doctor in terms that are technical or metaphoric, but the comparison of two medical systems has to find its way past the convenient terminology to the underlying theory which the doctor taps in making his or her diagnosis. Constructing a spirituality index would be a possible route for establishing comparisons.

The preference for the more spiritual quality over the more material is not an isolated choice, and each choosing has repercussions. If everyone in the community comes to prefer the spiritual, it will be seen more widely as more valuable, and the rest of the value system will adapt. This becomes a particularly influential pressure when the pattern of pure and impure situations works itself into the judgements on desirable employment and desirable marriage alliance. In Hindu India, for example, every kind of transaction is rated for its relative gain or loss of spirituality for the transactors. In the process a commonly agreed standard of ritual purity emerges. This is not first and foremost a matter for the philosophers, for the rating goes on in regular everyday thought and practice, and the philosophers justify or explain it afterwards.

According to McKim Marriott, the Hindu purity code provides a scale of values on which every kind of object can be graded. The spiritual end of the scale includes the more refined objects, the subtler media; the material end of the scale has the gross, lower, less refined, more tangible objects. Knowledge counts as subtler than money, but money is subtler than grain or land, whilst grain or land is not so gross as cooked food or garbage. Shedding blood or touching dead flesh is the grossest of all. The judgement of subtlety is not arbitrary, for it depends upon the possibilities of transformation.

Indian thought understands subtler substance-codes as emerging through processes of maturation or (what is considered to be the same thing) cooking. Thus subtler essences may sometimes be ripened, extracted, or distilled out of grosser ones (as fruit comes from plants, nectar from flowers, butter from milk); and grosser substance-codes may be generated or precipitated out of subtler ones (as plants come from seed, feces from food).

(Marriott, 1976: 110)

Every kind of transaction between castes is given a ranking, according to whether the giver is passing on gross or subtle substances to the receiver.

The caste ranking is like a ladder: higher castes are purer, and lower castes less pure. The offering and receiving of cooked food is the testing ground for claimed rank in the purity code. In this superb article Marriott analyses the strategies by which givers and receivers maintain or improve their position on the ladder of purity. It may seem remote and exotic to us here and now, but it would be self-deception not to recognize the Indian code as a consistently developed variant of the common model of classifying by degrees of spirituality.

To bring the topic nearer to home we can consider Pierre Bourdieu's (1979) theory of aesthetic judgement. For market researchers it has the practical advantage of predicting the choices made in different sectors of the French populace according to the distribution of what he called 'symbolic capital'. This is defined by contrast with economic capital. In practical terms symbolic capital means the investment made in training the judgement in matters educational, aesthetic, religious, ideological, metaphysical and so on. Basically symbolic capital can be represented as an investment in education that will yield income over time. It is possible to acquire it without special education if a person can establish a claim to intellectual or spiritual ascendancy. A preacher with direct revelation, or a healer, holds symbolic capital. It requires some kind of legitimacy, some kind of acceptability, but once it is there, it confers legitimacy on the judgements of its possessor. A church minister need not have years of seminary training to back his claims to a special relation with God, but if those claims are accepted in his congregation, the acceptance endows him with symbolic capital. The argument runs as follows:

1   Those who are well endowed with both economic and symbolic capital can call the tune for the reigning fashion in the arts. They are exemplified by the French *haute bourgeoisie*, represented in the liberal professions, in medicine and the law. In other words they form and conform to the tastes of the Establishment.

2   In contrast there are sectors of the population possessed only of economic capital, that is, new money without education. Lacking trained aesthetic judgement, and lacking social legitimation, their opinions on art have no legitimacy and tend to be greeted with derision. They are unlikely to be able to create a new movement of taste.

3   Other sectors have only symbolic capital and nothing else. They will be the radicalized intellectuals, the patrons of the Left Bank theatre, concerts and art galleries, writers and readers of critical theory and philosophical commentary. They love to mock the pretensions of the other culture-bearers, and define themselves against the established taste.

The trouble with Bourdieu's model is that it is so French. It is just as firmly rooted in the perspective of the nineteenth- and twentieth-century French bourgeoisie as the Hindu purity scale is rooted in India. For all that, his schematization of artistic taste is very suggestive for our problem about contemporary preference for the spiritual over the gross, and we can try to extrapolate from one to the other.

1   The well-heeled bourgeois élite endowed with both spiritual and economic capital would be expected to support Western traditional medicine. Why not? They are paying for the institutions which issue certification and which are intended to guarantee professional standards. Their judgement confers legitimacy.
2   The radical critique of the French Establishment flourishes among those who are strongest in symbolic capital and weakest in economic resources. We can treat the spiritual critique of modern medicine as parallel to the Left Bank critique of artistic taste. The same conditions that favour the radical critique would provide a sympathetic environment for the spiritual option.
3   As to those who have economic but lack symbolic capital, their being untrained in the enjoyments of refined taste might make them less enthusiastic for the spiritual end of the scale. At the least they are ill-equipped to judge the finer nuances. Some of them will certainly go for more robust choices, and we would not expect them to be candidates for a spiritualized medical theory.

Bourdieu has given us a kind of social epidemiology of where in a certain kind of society we should expect to find the demand for spiritualized medicine. But if we want to do research to test his model the question is how to exit from the tight framework of French culture. We need a more general model of where the taste for spiritual solutions is located. Bourdieu's argument implies that taste is always going to be harnessed to the struggle for hegemony in a particular community. He must be right: although good taste claims to rest on universal principles, it is always challengeable; the challenge comes from those who would subvert the established order, and the struggle is between them and those who want to manipulate it.

If we boldly draw an equivalence between the models of French good taste and Indian ritual purity we can see that in both cases the spirituality index has been harnessed to the social ranking of a hierarchical society, though inversely. For that reason neither case corresponds to what we are witnessing in respect of the demand for gentle solutions. For the movement which we are trying to understand is explicitly egalitarian. It is hostile to domination, and hostile to the authority of Western science. The contest polarizes two constructions of the medical practitioner: one whose authority depends on Western science and on the industrial democracy which produced it; and the other, who draws his authority from esoteric sources, from ancient cosmic knowledge.

Between one medical theory and another two views of reality are at issue. Traditional Western medicine and complementary therapy teach opposed theories about how the universe is divided up and where the parts fit together. We are dealing with two cultures. The question is not how two different realities become credible, since the reality is one. The question is about two different medical 'credibilities'. Some form of analysis more distanced, more abstract and generalizable will be necessary.

SICKNESS AS A RESOURCE

To talk fairly about what is credible and incredible in both forms of medicine the argument has to retreat to a level of abstraction which includes each as credible. Comparing two cultures, there can be no shouting down the other side, no privileging what is credible to one party and downgrading what is credible to the other. It would be cheating to take on board bits and pieces of the other view while rejecting various parts as unacceptable. To proceed by saying that chiropractice is acceptable but not acupuncture, aroma therapy but not reflexology, or the other way round, is merely exerting prejudice. A fair argument needs to be conducted on a common ground.

The cultural theory that I will apply starts from questions about solidarity. Culture is the way people live together. I would like to assume that it is extremely difficult for a group of people to live together in an organized way without force, and that heavy tactics of persuasion have always been used when any solidarity appears, even for a short time. Solidarity always needs explaining; long-term social harmony, I assume, is more difficult than short-term. As soon as I have proposed this minimum basis for my argument, I discover that, minimal though it is, it does not provide a common ground. My challengers will say that I am horribly biased in assuming that conflict is more probable than harmony; they will maintain that living together is no problem, so long as there is good will, kindness and self-denial. They might even add that complementary therapy is a means of achieving this desirable condition.

Immediately our search for a common ground for the argument has to begin again. Can we take it that solidarity is desirable? And that it is admirable when it appears? Is it safe to assume that we can recognize it when it is there? If we can agree that it is sometimes absent, then we may have some common ground for considering the forms of persuasion that produce variety among cultures.

This basis of comparison is fair to both sides. The argument will make the sick Londoner who is choosing complementary medicine equivalent to the African villager who is confronted by the reverse option. The choice is not between science or mumbo-jumbo, but choosing the traditional versus the exotic system, and in effect it means choosing between therapeutic communities. The African patient faced with the choice between the Christian missionary doctor with an exotic pharmacopoeia and the traditional diviner with his familiar repertoire is under the same sort of pressures as a Westerner choosing between traditional and exotic medicine. For minor ailments he can pick and choose separate remedial items without incurring censure, but if it is his own life or the life of his child that is at risk, his therapeutic community will take a strong line. He may have friends on either side of the divide, or choosing may involve him in a complete switch of loyalties. It is rather like religious conversion: if there is a strong political alignment dividing the two therapies, there will be political pressure not to convert to the other side. That is a good beginning for the anthropological approach.

The next step is to follow the monitoring that is going on in any community. Wherever there is illness, warnings are being issued, and informal penalties being threatened. When you define yourself as sick, you can escape censure for doing your work badly, being late, being bad-tempered, and so on, but the community which indulges the sick role also exacts a price: the sick person is excused remiss behaviour on condition of accepting the role, eating the gruel or whatever is classified as invalid food, taking the medicine, and keeping to the sick room, out of other people's way.

Having adopted the sick role, the patient cannot play any normally influential part. The patient is reproved for trying to go on working; if the patient complains of pain, the answer is that complaining is aggravating the condition and a more severely restricted diet may have to be prescribed; every complaint is met with potential criticism so that the patient ends by lying back and accepting the way others have defined the sick role. Dragging around looking tired, friends ask if the doctor has been called in yet, and if so, they want to know who, and are free with advice as to who can be trusted. It is a matter of pride for them if their favourite doctor is called, and there is a threat of withdrawn sympathy if it is one of whom they disapprove. These friends interacting with the patient, listening to symptoms and offering advice, form what the anthropologist John Janzen (1978) calls the 'therapeutic community'.

At the early stages of illness, there is some choice: either behave as if you are well or admit to being sick and bear the consequences. If the illness worsens and the invalid refuses the advice of friends and family, it is going to be difficult to ask for the neighbourly services or the loans of money on which lying in bed depends. The rival merits of traditional and alternative medicines are put to the test, not according to the patient's recovery but according to the negotiating of the sick role. The outcome will depend on the therapeutic community. For the sick person, the power of the medical theory counts for less than issues of loyalty and mutual dependability, unless he or she is completely isolated.

The background assumption is that any society imposes normative standards on its members. This is what being in society involves. Living in a community means accepting its standards, which means either playing the roles that are approved, or negotiating the acceptability of new ones, or suffering from public disapproval. The option for spirituality is a form of negotiation. But of course communities differ in the amount of control they exert: some are quite lax and standardization is weak; others exert ferocious control. In this perspective it would be interesting to know whether the persons who have chosen alternative therapy have also chosen a therapeutic community to support them with friendship and counsel.

For medical anthropology patterns of accountability are probably the most revealing of all the comparisons that can be made between different medical systems. It stands to reason that the more organization that is being attempted, the tighter the scheduling of coordination and the stronger the controls imposed. Where minutes count, the ambulance arriving half an hour after being called can be disastrous. Living in a tightly coordinated society can be itself a source of strain, and when the time factor starts to count more than the personal factor we glimpse a constraining set of circumstances. Bureaucratic mechanisms, lack of human concern, erratic interventions, episodic treatment, overcrowded clinics, unexplained delays, would diminish confidence in modern medicine and tempt towards the gentler therapies and their more regularly sustained treatments in the all-embracing cosmic scheme of things. These are the kinds of differences which cultural theory takes into account.

Starting from the idea that blaming and criticizing are essential social processes, anthropology recognizes that medicine is always under community control, and its justifications are always severely scrutinized. It is not just because health, life and death are important in themselves. All sickness and bodily impairment are grounds for demanding justification and so superb material for the blaming and justifying process. In the most extreme form, every illness affords scope for an accusation. If someone is sick, they can be accused of not taking proper care of their bodies. The sick person is not necessarily the one who is accused: if it is the children, the parents are accused, or the school, or the public sanitation. In this context of mutual recrimination the body is a medium for exerting control; pointing to a sick body is a potential threat against anyone who can be held accountable. Doctors do not normally think of sickness as grounds for accusations, and to some this view may be repellent. But we are not doing medicine, we are doing anthropology, and this is the most promising approach for comparing rival constructions of the therapist.

CORDON SANITAIRE AND HAND-WASHING

Medical anthropology has to be interested in the way that health is invoked to promote collaboration and rejection. Theories of contagion, for instance, serve as fences for keeping undesirables out. Leprosy, for example, without any well-founded diagnostic principles, was made a cause for segregating large numbers of the poor and landless in twelfth-century Europe. Bubonic plague was associated with immorality in the fourteenth century and everywhere believed to be brought by foreigners. If there were no danger from plague the people would have found other reasons for restricting travel and trade, but the disease afforded a powerful weapon for self-interested blaming and excluding. Since community always involves judgement and persuasion, the fragile human body is the political touchstone, and blame is the justification for exclusion.

Medicine is there, right in the middle of whatever issues are at stake, because human bodies are always at risk. But different kinds of societies allocate blame in different patterns. Medical anthropology ought to be able to describe these patterns: if the Punjabi patient has a sinking heart, what does he expect his community to do about it? If the Lele with pneumonia suffers from crossed-over ribs, what can be done to uncross them? In either case, what was the initial cause of the ailment? Who is to blame? The patient? Or the doctor? Or the mother-in-law? We will never get a satisfactory medical anthropology unless we demand to know the whole scenario. To describe diagnoses as if they were museum items is of no interest. We need a holistic context. According to what kind of blaming is going on, the role of the therapist will be differently constructed: to avert the finger of blame, to point it, or to attract it.

In some communities blame-averting techniques are well developed. Where social patterns are highly competitive and individualistic, no one who is engaged in the race for success will have time or resources to help the less successful. If the rewards for winning are great and the penalties for defeat heavy, failure will penalize the unsuccessful competitor's family as well as himself. In such a system failure is a frightening prospect; one who sees the scales turning against his own efforts will be apt to feel depressed and worried, become listless, lose appetite. His poor health is a reproach to his neighbours, but what can they do? A large loan can hardly be spared to one whose state of health suggests he is a bad risk, and when all the introductions to the powerful network are probably being used for family already. What is needed when it is impossible to cure the sickly neighbour is a ceremony that amounts to a show of sympathy while washing hands of responsibility. There are many examples of such hand-washing ceremonies.

The Gurage in Ethiopia used to have a theory that these symptoms indicate possession by a hungry spirit. When the friends and neighbours perform this ceremony the evil spirit is supposed to go away satisfied, allowing its victim to recover without further intervention (Shack, 1971). The therapist who plays the role of intermediary between malevolent spirit and human patient expects his fee. Who pays it? If the community is washing its hands of further responsibility, it might be reasonable to expect them to pass the hat round. If the patient does not recover, does he get called in again? Or is he sued for failure?

From the point of view of the community, the belief in bad spirits which upholds the hand-washing ceremony is relatively harmless, because no human gets blamed. The diagnostic theory sounds harsh, since the rite of exorcism does not help the patient in any of the material ways he needs to be helped. But comparatively it is benign, because neither the patient nor any of his enemies are made to carry the blame for his illness and the therapy enables everyone to get on with their lives.

Elsewhere responsibility for sickness has more sinister repercussions. Someone, neither the victim nor a hungry spirit, may be held responsible for insidious harm. This kind of diagnosis unleashes latent passions of fear and hate, and accusations are liable to tear the community apart. If this is the scene of diagnosis, then the therapist is constructed to point the finger of blame, and will presumably get paid by the accusers. In another type of society, the sick person is held to be suffering in punishment for his own delinquencies. For everyone except the patient this is a form of hand-washing in which the patient is made to carry the guilt of sickness. Though certainly unjust, in its social consequences this diagnosis supports the moral code. It is rough on the deviant, and much too kind to the sanctimonious busybody who is ready to suppose that the sick persons brought their troubles on themselves. But it has the great advantage that it lets the neighbours off the hook and does not set them against one another in angry recriminations.

It is tempting to dismiss the blaming and excluding processes of exotic or archaic medical diagnostics on the grounds that they belong to far away times and places. But blaming and excluding go on everywhere, and a medical anthropology that does not recognize this is trivial. The more highly organized the society, the more intense the accusing and inculpation. Modern medicine gives scope for prosecution whenever risks to health are incurred. So do not think that the approach via blaming is only relevant to distant tribes or far-off history. The accountability of modern medicine is highly institutionalized and the variations between nations are interesting in themselves.

The United States and the United Kingdom are two industrial nations which have inherited and share the same medical system. They can none the less differ in their medical practice according to the kinds of accountability to which the profession is subjected. In the United Kingdom doctors, ultimately, are answerable to the profession. Being struck off the list of accredited practitioners is a professionally exercised control; patients will turn to the BMA for redress before announcing their troubles to the press. In the United States the medical profession, which has a powerful political lobby, is relatively weak in policing its own members and more responsive to demands for accountability which come from the press and other lobbies. This makes a difference in judging what to do in a crisis. It is a pattern of accountability which makes for a more interventionist medical bias. In response to the media, the medical authorities have to be shown to be 'doing something', and to be more inclined to accept the 'worst case scenario'. For example, when a swine flu epidemic was predicted by Swiss researchers in 1976, the Americans, afraid of public censure, planned nation-wide prophylactic measures in case the worst should befall, while the British, more afraid of looking fools in the eyes of their professional colleagues and better protected from the media, were more sceptical about the evidence and decided not to undertake a massive inoculation campaign. In the end the worst did not befall and the more sceptical policy of the British turned out to be justified. But do not think that the doctors were acting on personal insights: they were socially constructed by the other institutions to which their patients and colleagues and they themselves subscribed.

CULTURAL BIAS

In applying the analysis of accountability to therapists in complementary medicine we are looking at the other end of the spectrum, not at those in positions of professional influence but at the general public making their choices about what kind of practitioner they prefer. To understand their liking for a spiritual medicine we need to set it in the whole context of their other preferences and attitudes to authority, leadership and competition. Cultural conflict is part of the explanation of their choice. We would expect people who show a strong preference for holistic medicine to be negative towards the culture in which the other kind of medicine belongs. If they have made the choice for gentler, more spiritual medicine, they will be making the same choice in other contexts, dietary, ecological as well as medical. The choice of holistic medicine will not be an isolated preference uncoordinated with other values upheld by the patient. Even labelling it more spiritual and claiming it preferable for that reason implies a latent protest against an established culture labelled materialist. The adepts need not be very articulate in reproaching modern industrial society for its violence and aggressive wars: they may tacitly disapprove the social inequalities, and the unequal distribution of wealth and income; they may privately deplore the destruction of earlier, more egalitarian social forms and cherish the traditions of more peaceful epochs. It is not necessarily an overtly political protest, nor does the person who holds these views need to articulate them in a more clearly political way. It is enough that they are saying that they believe that all bodies need a gentle therapy.

Anthropology can contribute to the understanding of movements in popular medicine by introducing the idea of conflicting cultural types. Two basic principles have already been introduced:

1 accountability as the context of community solidarity;
2 the role of illness in constituting the community.

We can add a third principle:

3 the principle of opposition: if one culture is to stay distinct, it needs to be defined in opposition to other cultures.

The idea is that in all their behaviour persons are continuously engaged in trying to realize an ideal form of community life and trying to persuade one another to make it actual. Little that is done or said is neutral, every aspect of living and all choices are tested in the struggle to make a cultural ideal come true. On this approach each cultural type is in conflict with the others and there is no line to be drawn between symbolic behaviour and the rest. Everything is symbolic and it is all heavily engaged. The same analysis that applies to the choice between religions applies to the choice of foods and of medical methods.

There are four distinct kinds of culture, no one of which can flourish in the conditions predicated for any of the others. The four can be quickly indicated by saying that one is based on hierarchy, and so in favour of formality and compartmentalization; one is based on equality within a group, and so in favour of spontaneity, and free negotiation, and very hostile to other ways of life; one is the competitive culture of individualism; and fourth is the culture of the isolate who prefers to avoid the oppressive controls of the other forms of social life. Any choice which is made in favour of one is at the same time a choice made against the others. The choices are made by the subjects of our study, and it is not our place to let personal preference between alternative ways of living bias the discussion.

In the social sciences a choice is treated as an individual matter, arising out of needs inside the individual psyche, and made to satisfy individual needs. The theory of culture, on the contrary, emphasizes the constitution-making capacity of individuals. We assume individuals are vitally interested in the kind of society they are living in. Any act of choice is also active in their constitution-making interests. A choice is an act of allegiance and a protest against the undesired model of society. On this theory each type of culture is by its nature hostile to the other three cultures. Each has its strengths, and in certain circumstances each culture has advantages over the others. And each has its weaknesses. But all four co-exist in a state of mutual antagonism in any society at all times.

It is important to appreciate that a person cannot for long belong to two cultures at once. The contradiction will be too difficult to live with, unless he or she can keep the contexts completely apart – home from office, leisure from home, etc. The cultures are in opposition to one another. Certain key preferences denote unambiguous alignment because they cannot be reconciled with their opposite. If the spiritual is chosen the material is ruled out. Formality cannot be practised at the same time as informality. Specialized functions are not compatible with general participation. No one can have both at once. Hierarchy disvalues equality, fervour opposes cool judgement, the excitement of crowds is at odds with the calm of order and the joys of solitude. We can think of more examples of cultural impossibilities: prepared sermons from the pulpit exclude spontaneous witnessing; standing rigidly to attention excludes rolling in the aisles; heterodoxy is opposed to orthodoxy.

Figure 1.1 illustrates in a general way the dynamics of opposed cultural bias. B to D is the diagonal of withdrawal or protest. B is the position of the Isolates, persons either who have been driven out of the running for power and influence by too strong competition, or who have chosen to keep out of the rat race, to avoid even trying to exert power. B, by definition, does not try to combine for opposition. The dissent is private, idiosyncratic, and not necessarily angry. The position at D is an organized dissenting Enclave, usually indignant against the abuse of power and wealth. Religious sects are the most familiar model of the Enclave culture. Though there is no expectation that cultural conflict in this corner will always focus on religion, the debate on principles of governance tends to raise the meta-physical stakes, so the more active the confrontation between the Establish-ment and the dissenting Enclave the more likely that spiritual values will be invoked sooner or later by the latter.

The use of schematic representation, as in Figure 1.1, is a technique for thinking about culture without indulging subjective bias. It explains how a bundle of preferences can be coded as either at the spiritual or the material

ISOLATES B   C HIERARCHY

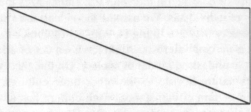

INDIVIDUALIST A   D ENCLAVE

Figure 1.1 General diagram of opposed cultural bias
Notes: AC diagonal – alliance of Individualist entrepreneurs with Hierarchists: cultural bias
        affirming authority.
        BD diagonal – alliance of Isolates at B with dissenting Enclave at D: cultural bias
        rejecting existing authority.

end of the spectrum. The theory is not deterministic. No one is forced by cultural pressures to choose one way or another. It does not even assume that people know what they want, but it does assume that they know what they do *not* like, and that they are realistic about their opportunities.

Moving between the different sectors is theoretically easy. Migrants, refugee victims of persecution or war and other displaced persons will be candidates for the corner of the Isolates. Historically many Enclaves have been formed by disaffected Hierarchists. Anyone who has rightly been classed as an Isolate may suddenly have the opportunity, for example, to own a street vendor's barrow or otherwise become a small-scale entrepreneur. Should his or her enterprise turn out well his formerly passive views about the universe will be likely to turn into the opportunism of the Individualist culture. Or failing such opportunity, there is nothing to stop a few Isolates from banding together and forming an Enclave, an ethnic, religious or therapeutic community. However, practice is different from theory, and in real life it is not always so easy to make the move between cultures, especially if friends see it as betrayal.

In any community there will be some sectors which are backing the structure of authority. The positive diagonal connects Individualism and Hierarchy as cultural allies. Both types of cultural ideal accept authority, leadership and domination. Individualists and Hierarchists alike believe that in the good society authority has to be exercised. Appropriate use of force poses no problem for them; they are much more liable to worry about subversion, arbitrariness and anarchy. By the same token, anything that they approve of will automatically be up for question by the cultures on the negative diagonal. By definition the Isolates will not be able to exert influence and will not expect to use force to attain their ends. The Enclavists will have combined together in protest against the domination of the mainstream society. Both the cultures on the extremes of the negative diagonal will be fertile ground for protest, and the obvious common ground they have for protest is the use of power.

For the people on the positive diagonal authority is, in principle, acceptable; in their different ways they are seeking to exert it; violence is disapproved if it is arbitrary, the subordination of animals is taken for granted. On the positive diagonal the coding of 'spiritual' versus 'material' values is weak. Like everyone else, they will recognize the contrast of spiritual, subtle, pure, refined, etc. as distinct from material, gross, impure, vulgar; the coding is going on all around them, but in this position the idea of 'materialist' will have a restricted meaning. It will be used not to refer to power and wealth, but to assess the relative value of work and leisure; commercial values will be coded more 'materialist' compared with ethics and art; spectator sports, boxing, wrestling, football, as less 'refined' enjoyments than literature, music, painting, sculpture. In Pierre Bourdieu's (1979) scheme of good taste this unradical, unpolitical coding will be coming from the sections of society who are well endowed with economic capital, ready to maintain and collaborate unproblematically with the social system as it presents itself.

On the other hand, 'spiritual' and 'pure' are more meaningful codings for Isolates and Enclavists, and for them 'materialist' conveys strong disapproval. They find themselves peripheralized in the mainstream society, unable to exert power, and without influence. On Pierre Bourdieu's scheme these will be the people who tend to be short of economic capital, but though they may not have symbolic capital in the form of education, they will have many ways of appropriating legitimacy to themselves. The preference for the spiritual is a grading and exclusionary device for use as a weapon in the war between cultures.

Set in the larger context which includes Indian vegetarianism and other ancient movements to cherish animal rights, it becomes easier to see why cultural alignments demand to be expressed according to a spirituality index. Wearing furs and eating meat, both of which license violence to animals, would come to symbolize corruption and abuse of privilege. All the products of violence stand at the impure or gross end of the spirituality scale, and would be associated with disregard for the environment and contempt for human values. If we can see how we ourselves develop definitions of pure and gross through classifications of food and clothes, we can see the spiritualist critique of medicine in the same perspective. Figure 1.1 shows how the conflict between two medical systems is part of the polarization of the two diagonals. On the negative diagonal, where it makes sense to be against harsh controls and exercise of authority, the option for spirituality is the more compelling.

CONCLUSION

Not everyone whose back is cured by a chiropractor or whose rheumatism is treated by a herbalist is committed to an explicit political programme. I do not know of any research that has inquired specifically about which sections of the population prefer spiritual versus material values. Colleagues who ask for quantitative evidence of the value of this cultural analysis must admit in fairness that the usual surveys are not made on this basis. They generally are content to draw up their comparisons on the narrow basis of choices between therapies. Or they try to find out if the adepts for holistic medicine are alienated or not. For stratifying the sample of the population used for surveys they use the usual demographic classifications. But political alignment is too gross a test for a subtle inclination to spirituality. And neither demography, nor income, nor education reveals cultural bias.

The movement for gentle therapies is a strong cultural undertow which does not show in answers to questionnaires about political or religious affiliation. We can specify what the kind of research that would test this admittedly speculative approach would need to do. First it would establish the local indicators for the 'spirituality scale'. This would have to be carried through the whole range of choices between gross and subtle, in food, clothing, decor, entertainment and politics. Choices of therapies would be expected to resonate with established cultural bias, and from this the role of the therapist could be predicted.

The argument suggests that holistic, spiritualized medicine is going to be a permanent feature of our cultural landscape. With the spread of industrialization a cultural audit would show that the negative diagonal is well populated. Industrial society tends to draw individuals out of their primordial contexts of loyalty and support and strands them in the sector of the Isolates. With economic recession the rejection of authority and polarization of political attitudes are likely to grow. Where Enclaves and Isolates flourish, the spiritual critique will continue to challenge the definitions of reality given by traditional Western medicine.

ACKNOWLEDGEMENT

I wish to thank the editors for their stimulating and salutory suggestions for improving the text, and also several others who were so kind as to read it for me and comment even more forthrightly: Susan Hogan, Magda Van Gompel and Eirlys Roberts.

REFERENCES

Bourdieu, P. (1979) *La Distinction*, Paris: Editions Minuit.
Herzlich, C. and Pierret, J. (1985) 'The Social Construction of the Patient: Patients and Illnesses in Other Ages', *Social Science and Medicine*, 20(2): 145–51.
Janzen, J. M. (1978) *The Quest for Therapy in Lower Zaïre*, Berkeley: University of California Press.
Krause, I.-B. (1989) 'Sinking Heart: A Punjabi Communication of Distress', *Social Science and Medicine*, 29(4): 563–75.
Marriott, McKim (1976) 'Hindu Transactions, Diversity without Dualism', in Bruce Kapferer (ed.), *Transaction and Meaning: Directions in the Anthropology of Exchange and Symbolic Behaviour*, Philadelphia: ISHI.
Sermeus, G. (1987) *Alternative Medicine in Europe: A Quantitative Comparison of the Use and Knowledge of Alternative Medicine and Patient Profiles in Nine European Countries*, Brussels: Belgian Consumers' Association.
Shack, W. (1971) 'Hunger, Anxiety and Ritual: Deprivation and Spirit Possession among the Gurage of Ethiopia', *Man*, 6(1): 30–43.

2 Autonomy, responsibility and midwifery

Calliope Farsides

At first glance the history of British midwifery in this century seems to have been largely one of battles fought between the medical profession, health care policy-makers and midwives, over who can best care for pregnant women and their babies. More recently the women themselves have joined the battle, and at times the engagements have been extremely heated.

The history of these encounters is well recorded elsewhere (Donnison, 1977; Martin, 1989), so this chapter will concentrate on one very specific issue, that is, the demand made by midwives for greater autonomy. This demand is in part born of the midwives' sense of being undervalued, and their frustration at not being able to fulfil what they see as their proper role. As such it is inextricably bound up with their pursuit of status and professional recognition. However, those who argue most convincingly for greater autonomy are those who also claim that pregnant and childbearing women would benefit were the midwifery profession successfully to secure fully autonomous status.

It remains to be seen whether greater autonomy for midwives is the *route* to an improved situation for themselves and the women for whom they care, or whether it is the *prize* they will be able to claim consequent upon certain important changes taking place.

PROFESSIONAL AUTONOMY

The concept of autonomy and the question of what it is to be an autonomous individual has interested a broad range of philosophers. The etymology of the word is useful in capturing the central idea behind the concept as, in the original Greek, *autos* means self and *nomos* means rule or law. The reference to rules and laws is significant as it allows us to distinguish autonomy from freedom or liberty which (in its simplest form) is concerned merely with doing as one wills.

Accounts of autonomy generally stress ideas of control and rational choice which do not have to be part of an account of freedom. I can be free but not autonomous, autonomous and unfree. However, in common with our understanding of liberty or freedom is the idea that to be autonomous is somehow valuable or good. Indeed, some philosophers would argue that the capacity to be autonomous is precisely what elevates human beings above other forms of life. If I am autonomous I am living a particularly valuable form of life, irrespective of the actual quality of that life in other respects; this is because I am in some morally significant sense determining the course of my life.

Interestingly, in its earliest usage within the Greek city-states, the term *autonomia* was applied to cities rather than to the citizens within them. A city was autonomous if its citizens had the right to make their own laws, as opposed to being ruled by some alien conquering force.

Claims to professional autonomy often begin with an analogous claim by the profession to self-regulation. A professional group is regarded as autonomous if it is found to govern its own professional activities and to exercise a significant amount of control over such matters as entry qualifications, education, practice rules and disciplinary procedures. If this can be shown to be the case in terms of the midwifery profession, it might follow that individual midwives can be said to benefit from the autonomy of their professional group in the same way as Athenians were thought to benefit from the autonomy of their city.

EDUCATION

In the United Kingdom, in order to qualify as a midwife an individual must complete either a three-year direct-entry midwifery qualification, or an eighteen-month specialist course after a three-year general nurse training (UKCC, 1991a: 8–14). The direct-entry qualification is a relatively new idea, but it has gained widespread support within the profession, lending credence as it does to the idea that midwifery is not simply a sub-discipline of nursing, but rather a discipline in its own right.

The midwifery profession voted unanimously to reject the Project 2000 initiative which now governs nurse training; however, this move had more to do with the desire not to be subsumed into nurse education than with any opposition to the educative principles involved. In many cases midwifery courses have been altered to come into line with the new-style nurse education which regards nurses and midwives in training as students rather than employee apprentices. The new-style midwifery courses usually include a broad range of subjects such as sociology, psychology, law and ethics alongside the more traditional disciplines, and many believe that the new generation is being educated in a manner far more conducive to the promotion of individual self-esteem and professional status.

However, there have been certain costs to the profession attached to the academization of midwifery education. Universities are now much more involved in the training of tomorrow's nurses and midwives, indeed they are often the institutions which award the new-style qualifications. Naturally, as the awarding bodies, the universities want some influence over the content of courses, and this necessarily means that the profession loses some of the control it had over the curriculum whilst education remained within specialized colleges and hospitals.

Having said this, the influence of the universities is restricted by the fact that all courses still have to be approved by one of the four National Boards of Nursing, Midwifery and Health Visiting. The validation procedure is extremely rigorous, but a recent change in policy means that, in England for example, the English National Board (ENB) has replaced its team of specialized officers with generalized education officers. Consequently a proposed midwifery course would no longer necessarily be scrutinized by members of the ENB with specialized knowledge and experience of midwifery. Many midwifery educators were concerned by this change, believing as they do that nursing and midwifery are not analogous, and that the important educational implications of the differences between them may not be recognized by those from a nursing background.

In response to changes such as these, officers of the Royal College of Midwives (RCM: the profession's trade union) have been quick to point out that a loss of control in the important area of education could easily threaten the autonomy of the profession. Picking up on their fears, the House of Commons' Health Committee Report on Maternity Services published in 1992 (hereafter referred to as the Winterton Report) clearly recommended that

> midwives should be afforded the same rights as all other professions over the control of their education. Whether in NHS or other institutions, midwifery studies should be afforded independent faculty status. Selection of candidates, curriculum planning, assessment processes and course validation must remain under the control of the midwifery profession. We would expect these principles to be upheld not only in the training establishments but also by the statutory bodies that set overall national standards for training and approve and monitor the courses.
>
> (Health Committee, 1992: 417)

In its response to this report the government stated that the statutory bodies for nursing, midwifery and health visiting should continue to 'follow the principle that midwifery practice should be determined, validated and monitored by the midwifery profession' (Department of Health, 1992: 2.20.7). To this end,

> Under the 1992 Act, the four national Boards of Nursing, Midwifery and Health Visiting are to be reconstituted, from April 1993, as smaller executive bodies directly appointed by the respective Secretary of State. Each Board will be statutorily required, in discharging its function, to take account of any difference in the considerations applying to the different professions (nursing, midwifery and health visiting). Ministers of the Health Departments have given an undertaking that the membership of each Board will include a practising midwife, either as an executive or non-executive member.
>
> (Department of Health, 1992: 2.20.8)

The importance of control over education is particularly apparent at a time when midwives are attempting clearly to define their role and gain the respect of fellow professionals. If midwives control their own education they can educate individuals to fulfil the role *as they define it*, and equip them with the skills *they* feel appropriate to advancing the profession.

REGULATION

Whatever control the midwives may exercise over their education, midwifery practice in the United Kingdom is ultimately governed by statute, whilst competency requirements are set by European Council Directive. At an individual level a qualified midwife must be registered with the United Kingdom Central Council for Nursing, Midwifery and Health Visiting (UKCC) if she wishes to practice. The UKCC is the profession's regulatory body, required by parliament to 'establish and improve standards of training and professional conduct' (UKCC, 1984: 43), and it is the statutory body with which individual midwives have most direct contact.

Prior to the establishment of the UKCC on 1 July 1983, three statutory bodies controlled the practice, education and training of midwives in the United Kingdom. These were the Central Midwives Board (England and Wales); the Central Midwives Board for Scotland; and the Northern Ireland Council for Nurses and Midwives. There were no significant differences between the various pieces of legislation governing the three bodies, and the UKCC claims to have inherited a well-established pattern for the control of midwifery education, training and practice dating back in parts to the beginning of the century.

The relationship between the profession and the UKCC is generally an untroubled one, which is encouraging given the common understanding of the UKCC's role as one of 'policing' the profession. As a registered midwife an individual is 'required to pay due regard to' the *Midwives Rules* (UKCC, 1991a), *A Midwife's Code of Practice* (UKCC, 1991b) and the *Code of Professional Conduct* (UKCC, 1992a), all of which are produced by the UKCC. These documents provide the midwife with the professional and ethical framework within which she is expected to operate.

The UKCC also publishes guidelines on specific issues, for example on *Confidentiality* (UKCC, 1987) and on *Standards for the Administration of Medicines* (UKCC, 1992b). On these more specific matters there is room for potential conflict, and it is perhaps inevitable that pronouncements upon such sensitive and complex issues will highlight divisions within the profession, and raise questions about the individual's autonomy within the group, an issue which will be discussed further below.

One way in which the UKCC clearly advances the autonomy of the professions it represents is by consistently promoting the view that nurses, midwives and health visitors are professional practitioners, worthy of the respect accorded to other professional groups.

> The perception of nurses, midwives and health visitors as professional practitioners is one which must not only be accepted by these professions, but by those with whom they work. To this end the Council will open channels of communication between the statutory bodies and other groups which will include the General Medical Council, professional organizations and trade unions and other specific groups and committees.
>
> (UKCC, 1984: 53)

This is an extremely important function given the way in which public perceptions of nursing and midwifery tend to support an old-fashioned view of a vocation rather than a profession. As will become apparent, the autonomy of the group is to a large degree dependent upon the recognition of its status by the other significant groups with which it interacts, most notably perhaps the medical profession.

DISCIPLINE

Whilst the UKCC is the national governing body, at a local level the activities of midwives are supervised by Local Supervising Authorities. These bodies appoint senior midwives to the position of Supervisor of Midwives, and pass to them the tasks of professional audit, support, advice and counselling. The Supervisor also has a legal duty to report alleged misconduct, with the final decision on these matters lying with the Professional Conduct Committee of the UKCC. In terms of discipline, therefore, most matters are kept within the profession.

The question of discipline is inextricably linked to issues of responsibility and accountability, and indirectly contributes to the attitude other groups will form towards the profession. If the midwifery profession is shown to monitor and respond appropriately to the misdemeanours of its members, its claim to be an autonomous self-regulating body will be enhanced. If, however, it appears to defend its members come what may, or to ignore serious lapses in standards, its position would be damaged.

PRACTICE AND POLICY

In terms of the autonomy to practise midwifery in the ways in which the profession itself sees fit, there can be problems. Within the National Health Service there is the problem that midwifery policy is too often determined by managers who do not come from a midwifery background. This is significant as it means that individual midwives may come up against policies which they are contractually obliged to implement, but which ignore or fall short of the standards set by their professional regulators.

In practice, the midwife will only be able to appeal to the *Code* in cases of gross conflict, and on a day-to-day basis there may be powerful reasons why the policy of the unit, hospital, trust or health authority will hold sway. This may, of course, become less of a problem as the changes in education equip a new generation to pursue management careers, and as midwife-managed units become more common, but the potential for conflict cannot be ignored.

It would appear from this brief survey that as a professional group midwives already enjoy some degree of autonomy when it is defined in terms of self-regulation. This is not to deny that certain areas of control which contribute to this autonomy need to be carefully guarded, for example education, and that others need to be developed further, for example policy-making. However, one soon realizes that issues of autonomy have to be considered at levels other than that of the professional body.

It has already been suggested that to understand a group as autonomous we have to know whether the autonomy of the group is sufficiently understood and respected by others. We also need to know how the individuals within the group understand their position, and how they are allowed to function, both in relation to the group and in relation to relevant out-groups.

In order to discuss these issues we require a fuller understanding of autonomy than the one offered so far, and we also need to engage in a careful investigation of the context within which this autonomy is claimed.

INDIVIDUAL AUTONOMY

Many definitions of autonomy have been offered by contemporary theorists, and it would be foolish to assume that they, let alone others, share a common understanding of the term they so readily employ. It has been claimed that

> I am autonomous if I rule me and no one else rules I.
>
> (Feinberg, 1972: 161)

and that

> A person is autonomous to the degree that what he thinks and does cannot be explained without reference to his own activity of mind.
>
> (Downie and Telfer, 1971: 301)

These definitions emphasize the direct sense of self-rule, and appear to equate autonomy with completely governing one's own actions, what has been called 'substantive independence' (Dworkin, 1988: 21–5). It has to be said that such definitions lock into many people's intuitive understanding of the concept, but the preceding account of midwifery as a profession shows that they are inappropriate in the present context.

Whilst midwives *as a group* might enjoy a significant degree of autonomy in the sense of regulating their own activities, the individual midwife is clearly governed, and sometimes constrained, by the rules and standards imposed by her membership of the group. In important respects she is ruled by someone, or something, else.

As a member of a professional body she is governed by the rules and regulations of that body, and her right to practise is dependent upon her behaviour remaining within the rules and standards set. As an employee she is subject to the rules and policies of her employer. Finally, as a member of a team she is subject to the commands of those placed in direct authority over her in her working environment, and she should be responsive to anyone within the team who places justifiable demands upon her.

Given these facts, a problem is immediately apparent. By placing a strong emphasis upon independence, we appear to make autonomy incompatible with any degree of direction or control by others. Indeed, such an individualistic account of autonomy even seems to work against the idea of cooperative ventures with others. It is obvious that the maintenance of professional standards requires that the individual midwife accepts at least the guidance, if not the control, of her professional regulators and colleagues. And, given that she will rarely operate alone in fulfilling her professional duties, we need to know that she can remain autonomous whilst fitting in with the practices and goals of her fellow team members.

We therefore need to explore a way of making autonomy compatible with concepts such as obedience and cooperation.

Those convinced of the importance of independence are not confident that this move can easily be made.

> The autonomous . . . man may do what another tells him, but not because he has been told to do it . . . by accepting as final the commands of the others, he forfeits his autonomy.

> (Wolff, 1970: 14, 41)

Accepting this view has a number of implications. Any formalized power structure which enables one individual to command the actions of another necessarily has to be interpreted as at least a potential attack on the subordinate's autonomy.

At one level, as previously mentioned, much of the midwife's activity is ultimately governed by statute and European directive, and she will have no direct involvement in the making of these rules. In this respect she is clearly governed by rules which are not of her making, but this need not necessarily mean that she obeys them simply because she has been told to do it. However, had she had a part in making the rules it might be easier to identify a different sort of reason for obedience.

It is notable that the UKCC *Code of Professional Conduct* (the regulatory document with which midwives will be most familiar) actively invites individuals to 'reappraise' the relevance of the Code, and encourages suggestions and comments which will be considered during the periodic review process. The Code is thereby presented as a living organic document with which the professional interacts, rather than a set of pronouncements carved on tablets of stone, and handed down by superiors. By allowing this degree of direct involvement and influence it is hoped that individual nurses, midwives and health visitors, will be prepared to make the standards set by the UKCC their own in the most significant sense available.

In the case of the Code, autonomy and rule-governed behaviour are reconciled by involving those who obey the rules in their formulation. However, because of the large numbers of people involved, and the complexity of some of the issues decided, it is not appropriate for all regulation of the midwifery profession to proceed on the model of a direct democracy. An alternative route towards reconciliation is to make the body enforcing the rules democratic in an indirect sense.

Since 1992, direct elections to the forty positions on the UKCC give all those who will fall under its governance an opportunity to authorize specific representatives to act on their behalf. This is a first step towards ensuring consent for the policies they will ultimately decide. In making their choices individuals will no doubt support the candidates whose views they believe to be right, or perhaps those they consider to be best equipped to perform the tasks set for them. In turn these candidates will seek to introduce measures acceptable to, or in the best interest of, their supporters. Thus, the regulations laid down should have a good chance of being accepted not simply because they are the commands of those in authority, but because they are acceptable to those who are required to obey them.

If this can be achieved, autonomy can be seen to be compatible with rule-governed behaviour for two important reasons. First, the rules have been made by individuals authorized to act on behalf of the person bound to obey them, and second, the rules are such that the individual could find an independent reason for obeying them, even if they were not commanded to do so.

In pursuing this line of thought some theorists have concluded that acting autonomously does not necessarily require even indirect involvement in rule-making, rather it involves acting from principles, or in conformity with rules, which we would consent to as free and rational beings. This is essentially a variation on the contractual model of rule, where the consent required is purely hypothetical and essentially retrospective. Our autonomy remains intact if we are regulated by rules we would have consented to (assuming that we are fully rational) had we been asked to do so.

This approach has both strengths and weakness. On the positive side it once again allows us to act in accordance with another's wishes or commands without forfeiting our autonomy. Our actions may be determined by principles set by others, as long as they are acceptable in some objective sense. However, real problems can arise in establishing what a free and rational being would consent to, or what is objectively rational.

One is reminded of the political philosopher Rousseau who asked that citizens participating in a direct democracy think only as citizens, and refer only to ideas of the Common Good and General Will (Rousseau, 1968: 59–62). Such demands leave no room for particular subjective interpretations or preferences. Rather, one is required to leave one's particular views behind, and to judge the principles in question, or the policy proposed, from a position of perfect impartiality, rationality and freedom.

Thus, by this theory, in order to ensure her autonomy the midwife must know that the rules and principles she follows, although set by others, would be consented to by her, in her role as midwife, given what counts as the common good in that context, and assuming her ability to discount considerations born of other allegiances and identifications. Given the difficulties involved in ensuring this outcome, it would appear wise to pursue another definition of autonomy as more appropriate in this context.

Luckily there are still further definitions of autonomy available, some of which attempt to tie the concept of autonomy closely to the idea of responsibility.

I and I alone am ultimately responsible for the decisions I make, and am in that sense autonomous.

(Lucas, 1966: 101)

This is a welcome step which is sometimes ignored when the concept of autonomy is employed as part of political or professional rhetoric. A claim for independence or control, which is so often at the heart of ideas of self-rule, must also entail the acceptance of responsibility if it is to carry any moral weight.

Responsibility can in turn be understood at a number of levels. I am causally responsible (at least in part) for those things I make happen, but I am not necessarily morally or legally responsible. Both in moral and legal terms we are prepared to make distinctions which are essentially based on the level of control I have over my actions, the intentions I hold, and what can reasonably be expected of me. The most complete case of responsibility involves a situation in which I am both causally and morally responsible for what I do, and legally entitled to be so.

As quoted above, the very definition of a midwife has at its core the idea of responsibility, and the UKCC *Code of Professional Conduct* also takes a clear line on accountability and professional responsibility. The introductory clause of the document unequivocally indicates that 'as a registered nurse, midwife or health visitor, you are personally accountable for your practice' (UKCC, 1992a: 1). In the UKCC advisory document *Exercising Accountability* the midwife is informed that

Accountability is an integral part of professional practice, since, in the course of that practice, the practitioner has to make judgements in a wide variety of circumstances and be answerable for those judgements.

(UKCC, 1989: 6)

The *Midwife's Code of Practice* states in its introduction that

Each midwife as a practitioner of midwifery is accountable for her own practice in whatever environment she practises.

(UKCC, 1991b: 1)

Clearly the professional body recognizes the importance of accountability, but further questions need to be raised. To whom is the midwife accountable, and to what extent is a linguistic shift between responsibility (which is our primary concern) and accountability permissible? Having set a standard of accountability we need to ask about the extent to which individual practitioners are willing, and/or able, to be responsible for their actions, which may not be the same thing.

To be accountable is to be answerable for one's actions to another person or body, in this case the midwives' professional body, her professional superiors (including doctors) and her managers. To be responsible is to be prepared to own one's actions in a fuller sense. It implies that I understand them as actions I have freely chosen to perform, and that because of this I will answer fully for the consequences of the action I take. To be accountable allows for the possibility of 'carrying the can' for actions which you were forced to take; to be responsible can entail vetoing demands which require you to perform actions you would not happily call your own.

Accountability can be demanded of those who have little or no real responsibility, but if individuals operate within a system which denies, or does not encourage them to take, personal responsibility for their actions, a valuable sense of autonomy might well be eroded. Even more fundamentally, if the system denies them a significant degree of control over their actions, it will be difficult to convince them that they should none the less remain responsible for their own actions. To be autonomous I need to be fully responsible, to be responsible I need to be in control of what I do, so some level of independence at least is called for.

If we accept the definition of a midwife adopted by the International Confederation of Midwives and the International Federation of Gynaecologists and Obstetricians (UKCC, 1991a: 2), the midwife will, by definition, be qualified to act in a responsible manner, and should be adequately equipped to offer justifications for her actions. Furthermore, according to the relevant European Community directive, she is 'entitled' to pursue the activities in which she has been trained.

> Member states shall ensure that midwives are at least entitled to take up
> and pursue the following activities.
>
> (European Community, 80/155/EEC Article 4)

Thus the midwife, assuming adequate education and experience, is capable of responsible action for which she can then be held accountable, and is entitled to fulfil her professional duties. However, the ability to do so does not ensure a willingness, nor indeed an opportunity, to take full responsibility in particular instances. To explore this issue we need to look at the context within which the midwife practises her particular skills.

THE CONTEXT OF CARE

At a practice level the degree of independence or control a midwife enjoys becomes much more dependent upon the context within which she operates. At one end of the scale the new breed of independent midwives operate outside the National Health Service, and the midwife enters individual contracts of care with the women she looks after. However, she will still be registered with the UKCC and thereby subject to its codes and rules. Community midwives and those involved in domiciliary schemes enjoy a certain independence by virtue of minimizing their contact with the hospital environment, whereas midwives operating within traditional consultant-led hospital units are those most obviously under the control of others.

As the result of deliberate government policy, in the present decade less than 2 per cent of births in the United Kingdom take place in the home (Health Committee, 1992: 14–34). The vast majority of births take place in consultant-led hospital units, and thus within the medically dominated hospital culture (Kitzinger and Davies, 1978). Given this fact, it is particularly important to find a way of explaining autonomy in terms of practice which does not initially depend upon substantive independence.

One feature of hospital culture is the existence of a clearly defined hierarchy which almost inevitably carries over into the experience of team work. A team can of course accommodate a formal hierarchy and still operate as a partnership characterized by cooperation, with a clear understanding of respective roles, and a common goal. However, when one looks at the average maternity team this is all too rarely an accurate characterization.

We must therefore look at this team very carefully, and assess how its dynamics contribute to, or militate against, the midwives' claim to autonomy, and the necessarily related issue of responsibility. For our purposes we can identify the core members of the team as the midwife, the mother and the doctor, who will be either an obstetrician/gynaecologist or a general practitioner.

Each of these groups is interested in the question of autonomy. It could be suggested that one group, the doctors, may wish to protect that which they have, whilst the other two groups are often devoted to obtaining more.

The previously quoted Winterton Report states with a note of regret that it often seemed that there was competition for control between these three groups. In responding to a statement by the Royal College of Midwives claiming a 'right' to practise in a system which made full use of their skills, the Committee were

> cautious about accepting that any one group has a 'right' to practise their profession which overarches the right of another group, or more importantly, might take precedence over the needs of mothers. We believe this has in the past been a way of thinking which has had adverse consequences for the maternity services.
>
> (Health Committee, 1992: 180)

It is important to understand what is at the root of this apparent battle for control if one is to understand claims for autonomy as something more than a tool of political rhetoric.

One factor which has helped to determine the current climate in maternity care is the success of the medical profession in taking control of the very definition and evaluation of childbirth (Farsides, 1992; Graham and Oakley, 1986). In doing so they have replaced the image of pregnancy and birth as a natural process generally proceeding towards a successful outcome, with the frightening image of a medical disaster waiting to happen. Consequently they have created a dominant role for themselves in a practice which had previously managed without them.

Since the late nineteenth century the success of maternity care has been evaluated in terms consistent with the medical model, that is, perinatal and maternal mortality rates, rather than women-centred evaluations in terms of satisfaction and health. In turn these figures have been interpreted largely in relation to medical practice as opposed to broader social and economic considerations. Thus, the conclusion that is drawn is that mortality falls when appropriate *medical* interventions are made, and appropriate medical interventions are defined as those which cause mortality rates to fall. The pessimism which accompanies any model of care which dwells on issues of mortality and morbidity means that it is all too easy to be convinced by the idea that a birth is only normal in retrospect.

Following on from this, women's choices of where to give birth have been restricted, and they have been actively steered towards hospital deliveries where medical interventions can most successfully be enforced. In 1970 a government committee report announced that

> We considered that the resources of modern medicine should be available to all mothers and babies, and we think that sufficient facilities should be provided to allow for 100% hospital delivery. The greater safety of hospital confinement for mother and child justifies this objective.
>
> (Quoted in Health Committee, 1992: 20)

In 1980 the government's Social Services Committee reporting on perinatal and neonatal mortality went even further in suggesting that

> We consider that the safety of the mother and baby in labour are of paramount importance and recommend that the labour ward should be regarded as an intensive-care area and that staffing and equipment be optimal.
>
> (Quoted in Health Committee, 1992: 23)

Although the first quote speaks only of making facilities available, in practice women have been actively discouraged from choosing venues other than a hospital for the birth of their child. Thus the Winterton Committee Report had to conclude that

> the choices of a home birth or birth in small maternity units are options which have substantially been withdrawn from the majority of women in this country. For most women there is no choice. This does not appear to be in accordance with their wishes.
>
> (Health Committee, 1992: 86)

The fact that almost all births now take place in hospitals, and even more significantly in consultant-led units, has a number of serious repercussions in terms of autonomy for both midwives and their clients. First, the doctor is operating on his home ground with all the security and control which this affords him. He can rely on the fact that the dominant culture within the hospital will reinforce his power and authority, and undermine that of the woman and the midwife. The doctor can dictate the level of intervention deemed appropriate because, having defined the context as medical, he can claim ownership of the specialized knowledge upon which decisions will be based. Furthermore, the fact that he bears ultimate responsibility for outcomes will make him cautious about sharing control with others.

The marginalization of the midwife is effectively achieved through restricting her role to 'normal' and 'low risk' pregnancies, whilst refusing to allow that most pregnancies fall under these headings. Even when a pregnancy is pronounced normal the consultant remains in control of important procedures such as admission to a hospital bed, or access to medical notes. As the Royal College of Midwives reports,

> We have had considerable difficulty in facilitating women having true choice over whether they wish to carry their own notes or not. . . . There are very few pregnant women who have the assertiveness skills sufficient to take on arguing with the medical staff. They often feel that their pregnancy care may be jeopardized in some way if they appear difficult.
>
> (Health Committee, 1992: 68)

It is also important to remember that whatever the particular arrangements within a specific hospital, the encounter between client, midwife and obstetrician is usually an encounter between two women and a man, and that it always takes place within a broader patriarchal system. It is not insensitivity to gender issues which has meant that doctors are characterized as male in this chapter. Figures supplied by the Royal College of Obstetricians and Gynaecologists confirm that the vast majority of obstetricians in the United Kingdom are still male, and this is particularly true at consultant level (RCOG, 1993).

One specific consequence of this is that those in control of the management of childbirth may have a limited understanding, and no experience whatsoever, of the process in question. Admittedly, few surgeons have experienced the procedures they perform on a daily basis, but one could argue that it is easier to work across from other examples in that context, than it is in the case of giving birth.

Finally, the medical model offers the doctor a particularly effective trump card. By emphasizing risk and danger the doctor has introduced a serious imbalance into any consideration of rights that might ensue. If we are told that on the one hand we have a woman's right to control the process of childbirth, or the midwife's right to practise her professional skills, and on the other we have the child's right to be born safely (maybe even its right to life), it is difficult to argue that they are rights of the same order. Indeed, one might be forced to admit that they are not properly comparable. If this is the case, the woman's claim to self-determination might be too easily trumped because it is played against the child's right to life and safety when in reality the risk of harm to the child is slight. Similarly, the midwife's claim to professional autonomy might be discounted as frivolous in comparison to issues of life and safety (de Gama, 1993: 114–30).

The preceding account raises a number of issues. On the one hand it would appear that an attack on the medically dominated definition of a good birth would contribute towards the possibility of beneficially altering the context within which midwives seek to claim their autonomy. What midwives must resist, however, is to become driven by 'territorial imperatives' (Health Committee, 1992: 25). The medical model cannot, and should not, be completely discarded, but rather the definition it provides should be extended to contain further non-medical elements. A first step towards achieving this is fully to involve all parties, including the recipients of care, that is, mothers, in the definition of a 'good birth'.

After listening to the views of many such mothers, and their representative bodies, the Winterton Committee prefaced its recommendations with a clear rejection of the medical model.

> We set out on this inquiry with the belief that it is possible for the outcome of pregnancy to be a healthy mother with a healthy, normal baby and yet for there to have been other things unsatisfactory in the delivery of the maternity care. Women want a life-enhancing start to their family life, laying the groundwork for caring and confident parenthood.
>
> (Health Committee, 1992: 3)

Becoming a mother is not an illness. It is not an abnormality. It is a normal process which occurs during the lives of the majority of women and can indeed be seen as a manifestation of health. It is physically very demanding and is a time when women are vulnerable in many ways. They require help and support during the process of being pregnant, giving birth, and postnatally and some of this, though not all needs professional help. In some circumstances the quality of the professional help is literally vital. But it is the mother who gives birth and it is she who will have the lifelong commitment that motherhood brings. She is the most active participant in the birth process.

(Health Committee, 1992: 4)

These are indeed noble sentiments but a word of warning must be offered against making too many general assumptions about 'what women want'. Women are culturally and individually diverse to an extent which denies us the possibility of offering a universal women-centred interpretation of childbirth. In fact, one might argue that the medical model is actually the one which most successfully locks into the common interests of all women – healthy baby, healthy mother.

Instead of assuming a homogeneity which does not exist, it is important to stress that a commitment to discovering 'what women want' involves getting to know individual women, and understanding the cultures and communities within which they are experiencing birth. The midwife could be a useful source of such information, as gatherer and cautious interpreter of women's stories.

It is also important to avoid jettisoning what is useful from the medical model. Considerations of safety are surely an important element of a good birth, and one which will feature in any woman's definition. It is even possible that at certain important stages they become the most important considerations, trumping other claims which contribute to a woman's overall satisfaction with the experience of childbirth.

Having helped to establish the definition of a good birth, the midwives can then contribute towards determining the best way of achieving this goal, and most importantly their role within the team. To develop this theme we need to return to the issue of autonomy.

When offering initial definitions of autonomy great emphasis was placed on being independent, being in control and not bowing to the will of others. Whilst this approach does much to protect individuals from those who might attempt to influence them without justification, it also works against the idea of allowing others to influence them within a cooperative and non-combative situation. As such, these definitions contribute to the 'territorialism' identified and criticized in the Winterton Report.

For this reason we moved towards definitions which allowed that a rational acceptance of control by others was consistent with remaining autonomous, and we stressed the need to accept responsibility for those areas in which one does exercise control. It is also worth stressing at this point that greater responsibility within the hospital, or indeed primary responsibility in a community setting, would have to carry with it legal responsibility for outcomes. This would potentially expose the midwife to the possibility of litigation should something go wrong, and for some this will be the cost of exercising greater autonomy.

None the less, such accounts allow for autonomy to be preserved even within a hierarchical or rule-governed context. An excellent example of such an approach to autonomy is that offered by the contemporary moral and political philosopher Gerald Dworkin. At first sight Dworkin's definition might appear unnecessarily theoretical.

> autonomy is conceived of as a second-order capacity of persons to reflect critically upon their first-order preferences, desires, wishes, and so forth and the capacity to accept or attempt to change these in the light of higher-order preferences and values. By exercising such a capacity, persons define their nature, give meaning and coherence to their lives, and take responsibility for the kind of person they are.
>
> (Dworkin, 1988: 20)

However, it can soon be translated into more everyday language. The distinction between first- and second-order desires and preferences is one often employed by philosophers. Essentially our first-order desires are those we feel most immediately and instinctively, for example the desire for a stiff drink at the end of the day. Second-order desires are immediately more reflective and are formed not with reference to our basic impulses, but rather in relation to rational principles or preferences we might hold.

So, for example, whilst I have a first-order desire to gulp down a large gin and tonic, I may also have a second-order desire not to rely on alcohol as a prop. Although my autonomy does not depend on the second-order preference winning out on every occasion, it is dependent on my critically assessing my first-order desire in the light of it. I may well decide that one gin and tonic does not conflict with my desire to remain independent of alcohol, but I need to be in a position to make this evaluation to be judged autonomous.

This is the basic concept with which Dworkin works, but what is most interesting in the present context is the new perspective his definition permits on the issue of independence as it relates to autonomy. On Dworkin's account it is possible to hand over a significant degree of control and responsibility to another person and remain autonomous with respect to the issue in hand. Let us see how this would work within the midwifery team.

Using Dworkin's first- and second-order distinction it is apparent that each of the groups represented within the midwifery team has a strong first-order desire for independence, power and control and that this is often voiced in terms of claims to autonomy. However, on reflection, they would be forced to admit that in certain situations these objects of desire have no instrumental value. Furthermore, the desire to exercise power or control in a situation where one is unequipped to do so, or to claim independence when one cannot look after one's own or another's interests, could be seriously counter-productive.

As a group the maternity team should share one fundamental desire which is that the management of the pregnancy and childbirth be satisfactorily achieved (satisfactorily having been defined in a manner acceptable to all parties). Unless the exercise of greater power and control is an appropriate means to this shared goal, the desire for such things may have to be trumped, or at least tempered, by considerations more appropriate to securing a successful outcome.

As previously stated, if one decides to hand over a degree of control, forgo some independence, or give another power to act on your behalf, one may still be considered autonomous if the decision was based on a rational evaluation of the reasons for doing so. The danger is that those to whom control or power is transferred may take advantage of the transfer, and attempt further paternalistic behaviour which is unwarranted.

There is obviously legitimate scope for a division of labour within the team. A woman should not feel that she has to be in control of the whole process of pregnancy and childbirth in order to protect her autonomy. She will benefit from professional guidance, and in some situations it will be vital that those with expert knowledge take control of the situation. The midwife will be able to fulfil the primary role in offering support to the woman, but there will be certain procedures for which she has not been trained, or situations in which she feels unable to take responsibility – on these occasions the doctor will be able to assist. Were we to work towards a de-medicalization of the process, and broader definition of a good birth, he might be forced to accept that his role could be safely limited.

As long as each party judges any limitations placed upon them as appropriate to the end they share, or any hand-over of control as justified by the *true* facts of the case, autonomy will not be threatened. This would then leave the way clear for the team to develop policies directed towards a cooperative fulfilment of their relative tasks, and release them from the burden of fighting to make the process their own.

The midwife can facilitate this development in a number of important ways, some of which have already been discussed. She can continue to question the dominance of the medical model and the over-tendency to use the labels 'at risk' and 'abnormal' in relation to childbirth. To be in a position to do this she will need to refer to reliable research and clinical audit so that she is armed with facts rather than beliefs and opinions which can more easily be ignored. Midwives should produce such research, and having done so they should pay due regard to the results. It has been shown that midwives give less credence to research which has been carried out by their peers rather than by doctors, and this tendency has to be extinguished (Hicks, 1992).

The midwife can try to resist the temptation to collude with the medicalization process beyond the level demanded by reasonable considerations of safety (Bergstrom *et al.*, 1992). She can also support those women who reasonably request a home birth, and accept the greater responsibility which goes along with moving her practice outside the hospital setting.

Having said this, midwives must also guard against simply replacing the medical model with one of their own making. Although there is an argument to suggest that a greater commitment to post-registration clinical training would help them to attack the doctors' claim to specialized knowledge, they must also continue to consult and observe the women they care for, and acknowledge and incorporate the diversity of their non-clinical views.

This role of advocate will not be easy. As in any other situation, the voices that are most easily heard are those of the educated white middle class, but the midwife must listen out for different voices, and help to articulate the requests that they make. Sometimes these voices will have been silent, not because they have nothing to say, but because they are particularly disempowered by the situation within which they are required to speak.

In terms of activity at a professional level, the UKCC and the RCM must continue to support and promote the autonomy of individual midwives, and of the profession as a whole. Where appropriate they must protect their group's independence, but they must be careful to remember that an adequate definition of autonomy demands much more of them than this. Being autonomous is also about being competent and responsible, and the maintenance of high professional standards is an important contributory factor to such capacities.

The extent to which the individual midwife's autonomy is respected by others is eventually outside the profession's control. Government policy will continue to determine the context within which care is delivered, and the attitudes of the medical profession will always be an important consideration. Doctors cannot be forced into re-evaluating their relationship with the midwives, but the professional bodies can attempt to facilitate such a process.

A WAY FORWARD

In this chapter it has been suggested that issues of autonomy need not necessarily boil down to issues of independence and control. It has also been suggested indirectly that maternity care in this country will only improve if all parties involved resolve to eschew territorial warfare, and concentrate instead on the fostering of mutual understanding and recognition.

A midwife who clearly understands herself as a member of a team will not make her own autonomy her primary goal, instead she will focus on perfecting her contribution to the team's work and thereby she will earn her autonomy. She will also respect the autonomy of others, particularly that of her clients, and she will seek to promote it where appropriate – sometimes by forfeiting her own independence.

It seems clear that the individual midwife will protect her autonomy not through territorial battle but rather through developing her skills and proving her worth. Essentially it will be a reward for undergoing her education, demonstrating good practice, and accepting professional responsibility. A good midwife will enable others within the midwifery team to hand over control to her without them feeling that their own autonomy is in any way threatened. Similarly she will acknowledge the skills of others, and where they are more equipped (or have more right) to manage the situation, she, too, will stand aside without believing that her autonomy is diminished.

ACKNOWLEDGEMENT

I would like to thank Greta Beresford, Rachel Clarke and Bobby Khan for the help they gave me in preparing this chapter. Needless to say, the views expressed and any mistakes made are all my own.

REFERENCES

Bergstrom, L., Roberts, J., Skillman, L. and Seidel, J. (1992) '"You'll Feel Me Touching You Sweetie": Vaginal Examinations during the Second Stage of Labor', *Birth*, 19(1): 10–18.

de Gama, C. (1993) 'A Brave New World? Rights Discourse and the Politics of Reproductive Autonomy', *Journal of Law and Society*, 20(1): 114–31.

Department of Health (1992) *Maternity Services*, Cm 2018, London: HMSO.

Donnison, J. (1977) *Midwives and Medical Men: A History of Interprofessional Rivalry and Women's Rights*, New York: Schocken.

Downie, R.S. and Telfer, E. (1971) 'Autonomy', *Philosophy*, 46: 293–301.

Dworkin, G. (1988) *The Theory and Practice of Autonomy*, Cambridge: Cambridge University Press.

Farsides, C. (1992) 'Body Ownership', in S. McVeigh and S. Wheeler (eds), *Law, Health and Medical Regulation*, Aldershot: Dartmouth.

Feinberg, J. (1972) 'The Idea of a Free Man', in R.F. Dearden (ed.), *Education and the Development of Reason*, London: Routledge.

Graham, H. and Oakley, A. (1986) 'Competing Ideologies of Reproduction: Medical and Maternal Perspectives on Pregnancy', in C. Currer and M. Stacey (eds), *Concepts of Health, Illness and Disease*, Oxford: Berg.

Health Committee, House of Commons (1992) *Maternity Services Second Report*, London: HMSO.

Hicks, C. (1992) 'Research in Midwifery: Are Midwives Their Own Worst Enemies?', *Midwifery*, 8(12): 18–22.

Kitzinger, S. and Davies, J.A. (eds) (1978) *The Place of Birth*, Oxford: Oxford University Press.

Lucas, J. (1966) *The Principles of Politics*, Oxford: Oxford University Press.

Martin, E. (1989) *The Woman in the Body*, Milton Keynes: Open University Press.

Rousseau, J.J. (1968) *The Social Contract*, ed. M. Cranston, Harmondsworth: Penguin.

Royal College of Obstetricians and Gynaecologists (1993) *Fellows and Members by Country of Residence*, list supplied on request.

UKCC (1984) *Annual Report for the Year 1983–84*, London: UKCC.

UKCC (1987) *Confidentiality*, London: UKCC.

UKCC (1989) *Exercising Accountability*, London: UKCC.

UKCC (1991a) *Midwives Rules*, London: UKCC.

UKCC (1991b) *A Midwife's Code of Practice*, London: UKCC.

UKCC (1992a) *Code of Professional Conduct*, London: UKCC.

UKCC (1992b) *Standards for the Administration of Medicines*, London: UKCC.

Wolff, R.P. (1970) *The Autonomy of Reason*, New York: Harper & Row.

3 Quacks

An unconscionable time dying

Roy Porter

The long survival of quack doctors presents a historical puzzle. If, as we have endlessly been told by doctors and historians alike, they were frauds, crooks and incompetents, why did the sick continue to draw upon their services? Gullibility and lack of other options are possible answers, but it seems much more plausible to suggest that irregulars commonly established personal therapeutic relations with their patients that gave at least psychological support to sufferers and often made good use of the placebo effect.

I explore this possibility below, looking at the history of irregulars from the seventeenth century onwards. I suggest that quacks managed to establish a variety of fruitful patient–doctor relations; that they paid special attention to the 'public relations' side of the therapeutic encounter; and that they were sensitive and attentive to consumer demand – as they had to be.

INSIDE AND OUTSIDE

Quacks do not form a natural species; they are an artificial category, existing in the eye of beholders attuned to regular medicine and its claims. Like religious heretics and other 'deviants', they have been stigmatized as 'outsiders' by those on the 'inside', in this case the medical establishment. Of course, some doctors, like certain heretics, have always wanted to be lonely eminences, thumbing their nose at the Establishment. Yet the point is that the distinction between 'inside' and 'outside', 'central' and 'marginal' practitioners, assumes its great significance only because 'insiders' have drawn up exclusive boundary lines. For this reason, terms like 'fringe medicine' 'marginal medicine', and 'alternative medicine' are apt descriptions of quack practices: the sociological terms convey the fact that certain medical practitioners have been empowered to draw upon legalized professional authority and sanctions, whereas others have often been on the receiving end of these punitive sanctions, and have had to make their way in the world by other means.

Historically it makes more sense to distinguish between orthodox medicine and quackery on the grounds of legal and professional inclusion and exclusion than on any objective judgement regarding the quality of treatment given, its scientific standing, or its success rate. It would be simplistic and misleading to take it for granted that official medicine has always been skilful whereas fringe medicine has been incompetent or fraudulent. At least before the widespread adoption of anaesthetics and antiseptic surgery from the nineteenth century or the development of sulfa drugs in the 1930s and antibiotics from the 1940s, the treatments administered by official medicine – traditionally, bleedings, purgings and vomits – probably did no more or less harm than those of fringe medicine. Of course the regulated orthodox, medical professions are unlikely to have housed *deliberately* fraudulent practitioners, whereas fringe medicine has always had its black sheep, from the huckstering mountebanks frequently satirized in seventeenth-century plays and satires, to the monstrous 'toadstool millionaires' who swindled the public with patent medicines in nineteenth-century America. Yet against this, orthodox physicians have never disdained fat fees, although disavowing the mercenary relations of business.

Nor can we distinguish between orthodox and fringe medicine on the grounds that official medicine has always been 'rational' and 'scientific' in its methods, whereas quack medicine has fallen back upon magic, showmanship and psychological deception. After all, orthodox medicine has possessed its own potent rituals. The gentlemanly bedside manner, the cultivation of literary graces, the use of Latin as mumbo-jumbo, the ancestor-worship of Hippocrates and Galen, and exclusive access to the occult wisdom of humours or urine-gazing – all these have created the aura of the medicine man *within* the profession at least as much as the traditional quacks' alligator, black cats, snakes or neologisms. In an age in which there was no reliably efficacious *materia medica*, psychological soothing or the placebo effect – whether it came from orthodox or fringe medicine – must have been a major component of successful therapy.

In many respects, therefore, it would be inaccurate to differentiate between orthodox practitioners and quacks on scientific and medical grounds. Many marginal doctors had extensive medical training before marketing nostrums or developing their own unorthodox medical aetiologies and therapies. From the sixteenth century onwards, no one but a graduate of Oxford, Cambridge or Trinity College, Dublin, could become a Fellow of the Royal College of Physicians and officially practise physic lucratively in London. Hence ambitious and well-trained medical graduates of Glasgow or Edinburgh, excluded from fashionable general practice and hospital consultancies in London, had to seek their fortunes towards the medical fringes. After the mid-eighteenth century, many set up as specialists in treating particular conditions, such as diseases of the ear, eye or throat, or as obstetricians. For this they were liable to be roundly abused as quacks by leaders of the colleges: for long the 'specialist' was regarded as suspect in orthodox eyes; only gradually did he win the prestige he now enjoys.

The boundaries between fringe and core medicine have been contingent, fluid and negotiable. Certain fringe practitioners have always been keen to join the Establishment or at least to bask in its prestige. Some have sought respectability by setting up institutes. The Perkins family, late eighteenth-century promoters of metallic tractors like tuning forks that 'cured all' by a kind of mesmeric power, set up the Perkineian Institute in London. In the 1830s, James Morison set up a headquarters on the Euston Road called 'The British College of Health' to promote the sales of his panacea pills.

Some fringe practitioners, long anathematized by orthodox medicine, have acquired respectability and acceptance in time, partly through public patronage. Inoculators against smallpox were initially held at arm's length in France, but finally found acceptance. In England, advocates of 'moral therapy' for the mentally ill began to win acceptance in the first half of the nineteenth century, despite opposition from physicians committed to organic approaches and psychotherapies. Here, as often, questions of monopoly and licensing were to the fore. Many of the early 'moral therapists' were not trained and certificated medical men. Certain physicians claimed that only the medically qualified were fit persons to run asylums.

Orthodox medicine has often assimilated a fringe practice rather than lose patients *en masse* to marginal medicine. This usually happens through an astute filtering process: the metaphysical claims of the fringe practice are abandoned, while its practical techniques are absorbed. As a system of character analysis and of diagnosing mental disease, phrenology initially met powerful opposition. But once, from the mid-Victorian period, some of its more dubious claims – such as the identification on the skull of over thirty seats or faculties – had been played down, phrenologically inclined medical men became more acceptable. Watered-down phrenological beliefs, for example, the notion that the brain was the organ of the mind, soon themselves became medical orthodoxy. In a similar way, the metaphysics of mesmerism (the idea, originally advanced by Franz Anton Mesmer, that the universe was filled by a circulating 'animal magnetism') lost credence, but its technique of hypnotism became therapeutically used, for instance on patients undergoing dentistry or surgery. In short, the distinction between quackery and orthodoxy is essentially social. Quacks are those doctors excluded from professional power and privilege.

From medieval times all major European nations developed systems of medical licensing, policed by the upper echelons of the medical profession, and ultimately sanctioned by government. During the Renaissance era, the larger Italian towns in particular possessed official medical bureaucracies, with extensive regulatory powers over public health and hygiene. In the eighteenth century in France and the German principalities the idea of 'medical police' became popular: the state would empower authorized practitioners to take control over health matters such as quarantine or the licensing of apothecaries. Orthodox medical men were given ever larger public health powers within the state in the nineteenth century. Furthermore, from the Middle Ages, medical men had operated guilds and corporations policing entry into the profession. In these ways, an oligarchic inner core to the profession grew up, exercising a near monopoly of access to promotion, power and favour.

Incorporations of physicians and surgeons always sought a closed shop on the grounds of maintaining professional standards. Numbers were kept small, and so fees remained correspondingly high. Keeping numbers at the top small was certainly effective in stigmatizing and marginalizing other practitioners. But it was very ineffective as a way of *suppressing* unorthodox practitioners. This is partly because there never were enough privileged practitioners to meet the demand for medicine services. This was so especially in outlying parts far from capitals and other cities which housed fashionable physicians. Thus there were few well-trained physicians in the French countryside in the eighteenth century. As one disapproving physician commented:

> There is only one physician in the entire district of Josselin. Unless I am wrong, everyone is a physician: there is no one, of either sex, who does not meddle with giving advice to the sick, prescribing for them, or forbidding them to accept the most essential treatment and the most energetic remedies used in medicine.

Ordinary people have either had to take to self-medication or use quacks.

Many were not able to afford élite medicine. Patent medicines were cheaper, and quacks made it their business to make an appeal to common people whereas orthodox medicine has stood off. 'The rich and the great', commented the *Gentlemen's Magazine* (XVIII, 1748: 346),

> will seek relief from the regular physician, and true-bred apothecary; for whom provision is made in the college dispensatory. – But the majority of mankind (in hopes of saving charges, and on a presumption of surer help) are apt to resort to the men of experience, as they are called, whose remedies they are induced to think, from their advertisements (so often repeated, and at so great expense) have been successful in the cure of the several distempers for which they are calculated.

Out of genuine philanthropy or a shrewd business sense, quacks often made a show of dispensing free to the poor and the unfortunate. In the 1730s, Joshua Ward, who made a fortune out of his 'Pill and Drop', dispensed free to the poor. He kept 'poor houses' in Pimlico which were 'crowded with objects of charity to whom he always gave with the greatest humanity his medicines'. In any case, Establishment medicine has never commanded complete confidence. Its record of cures in previous centuries was unimpressive. In crucial matters of life and death, patients have always wanted to shop around.

In eighteenth-century England, when Prime Minister Sir Robert Walpole found no relief in orthodox medicine for his stomach ailments, he had resort to Joshua Ward's Pills (which were claimed to dissolve kidney stones). Even physicians resorted to unorthodox practitioners. Sir Hans Sloane, a leading physician in early eighteenth-century England, had a niece with a spinal deformity. When orthodox treatment failed, he called in the bone-setter and manipulator Sally Mapp, who worked a cure.

Partly for this reason, even those who could afford orthodox medicine have often tried quack remedies. There was nothing to lose. Furthermore, quack therapies have often possessed a fashionable novelty. Sometimes they have been less disgusting and severe than orthodox medicine's artillery of purges, bleedings and vomits.

Certain fringe practitioners, like certain evangelical preachers, have always drawn a following from high society. This is partly because of the lure of variety. Wealthy invalids with time on their hands would want to try novel treatments. In Central Europe, Viktor Preissnitz's health-farm hydrotherapy became fashionable in the nineteenth century. In one year his patients were said to include one royal highness, one duke, one duchess, 22 princes and princesses, 149 counts and countesses, 88 barons and baronesses, 14 generals, 53 staff officers, 196 captains and subalterns, 104 high and low civil servants, 65 divines, 46 artists and 87 physicians. Hypochondriacs and valetudinarians were often flattered by the assiduity and attention they received from certain polished fringe doctors. Unorthodox practitioners such as Franz Anton Mesmer and James Graham in the late eighteenth century were skilful showmen and actors who, when demonstrating the principles of their therapies at private *séances*, would give dazzling and spell-binding performances, equal to a Keane in the theatre, a Davy at the Royal Institution, or a Whitefield in the pulpit. Graham, an advocate of vegetarianism, mud-bathing and sexual rejuvenation, combined a marvellous theatrical touch with a sure grasp of audience psychology. In the words of the contemporary German writer W.D. Archenholz, he had

A perfect knowledge of the human heart, the success which attended his experiments proves that he has calculated with judgement. He has too much sense to be suspected of being a dupe to the occult science which he professed and must therefore be classed in the list of cunning and politic adventurers. . . . Nothing indeed is more superb than his Temple. Electrical fire, managed with judgement ascended in radiating streams: transparent glasses every different colour chosen and placed with taste, rich vases filled with the purest perfumes, which gently awaken desire, filled the soul with a soft langor. . . . The more that this holy of holies began to be visited, the more did this sagacious high priest add to the voluptuous magnificence of the place!

What is more, quacks such as Mesmer and Graham actually addressed themselves, more than most physicians, to those very problems that were the real ills of high society: *ennui*, anxiety, hysteria, sexual incompatibility, depression and nervous disorders. Their therapies, with their mixture of sympathy, suggestion and titillation, may have created a more relaxed atmosphere within which nervous ailments could be handled.

THE MEDICAL MARKET

The medical profession has been monopolistic without actually possessing a monopoly. The irony is that fringe practitioners were forced out into the market-place, at the very time when – with the development of capitalism – the market-place was the very springboard to expansion, success, wealth and fame. The medical profession practically ensured the prosperity of the men they proscribed.

Licensed medical men traditionally based their standing in the public eye on their corporate professional credentials: they have had behind them accredited education and certification; they have followed the official pharmacopoeia and medical ethics; the medical corporations have undertaken to purge themselves of incompetence and malpractice. The individual physician's authority has been that of the profession. By contrast the unlicensed practitioner's name came entirely from his standing with the public, not his peers. He was forced to act like a tradesman. He had to sell his wares in the market, creating by his own person whatever trust he could, and appropriating what sources of authority were within his grasp. The success of quacks has therefore been simply their success as tradesmen. They have not missed an entrepreneurial trick: in fact, they have pioneered many of them.

Many have been smooth-tongued showmen. Some, such as the Prussian influenza-curer Gustavus Katterfelto in the 1780s, exploited a penumbra of magic, wonder and wizardry: black cloaks, snakes, black cats, fuming potions and electrical sparks. Mountebanks traditionally toured accompanied by monkeys and zanies. Some sought status in the public eye by making the most of being – or pleading to be – foreign and exotic. The 'Chevalier' Taylor, the eighteenth-century eye specialist, lectured in pidgin Latin which he confidently but inaccurately described as 'The True Ciceronian'. Some assumed authority by adopting phoney titles, calling themselves 'Doctor' though they had no degree; Thomas Holloway, the nineteenth-century patent medicine king (and founder of the Royal Holloway College), styled himself 'Professor'. Others sought credit by dropping the names of the powerful and famous. Bottles of 'Daffy's Elixir' had a label stating that 'The Elixir was much recommend to the public by Dr King, Physician to King Charles II, and the late learned and ingenious Dr Radcliffe.' Joshua Ward, the marketer of the famous 'Pill and Drop', won himself fame and public confidence after putting George II's dislocated thumb back in place. He also received the testimonies of famous men. The novelist Henry Fielding admitted his 'obligations to Mr Ward. . . . I am convinced that he omitted no care in endeavouring to serve me without any expectations or desire of reward' (1755: 197). Partly as a result, Ward got official backing for his medicines. In 1753 his fever powders were ordered for all ships in the British Navy – twenty-five powders being allowed for each ship in the Channel Fleet, and seventy-five for each vessel in the West Indies.

At least up to the mid-eighteenth century, most quacks did their business through personal sales. Some had shops. Most, however, were itinerant. The travelling salesman had the aura of mystery. He was more elusive to the authorities. The mobile quack did not need to take responsibility if his cures failed; he set little store by regular customers. Having saturated one market, he could move on. This was important when the fringe practitioner was offering specialist services. Even as late as the end of the eighteenth century large country market towns in England and France did not have a permanent specialist tooth-drawer. Such a man would visit perhaps for a month a year, straightening teeth, supplying false ones, performing capping. Emergency extraction could always be done by a farrier or a barber. Itinerant quacks often sold other commodities as well as medicines: books, fancy goods, toiletries, tea.

From the eighteenth century, however, quacks increasingly plugged into the widening capitalist market. The growth of literacy and the rise of the newspaper permitted advertising on a large scale for the first time.

The Widow READ, removed from the Upper End of Highstreet to the *New Printing-Office* near the Market, continues to make and sell her well-known Ointment for the ITCH . . .

announced the *Philadelphia Gazette* on 19 August 1731. Similarly in the *Boston News-Letter* for 26 November 1761, Charles Russell of Charlestown announced that 'At his Shop at the Sign of GALEN's HEAD opposite the Three Cranes and near the FERRY' he had for sale, imported on the latest ships from London, 'Drugs, and Medicines, Chymical and Galenical', and certain patent medicines: Bateman's and Stoughton's Drops, Lockyer's, Hooper's and Anderson's Pills, British Oyl and Daffy's Elixir.

Newspaper advertising multiplied the potential market for quack preparations several thousandfold at a stroke. In eighteenth-century England, the medicines in question – such as Daffy's Elixir, or Dr James's Powders – were usually sold retail by the newspaper publisher. In the next century, capitalizing on the cheap and reliable postal service, and most notably in America, clients were urged to send money to the quack doctor's residence, depot or clinic. The public might prefer discreetly anonymous buying, especially when purchasing abortifacients or cures for impotence.

Quacks showed great flair in advertising techniques. Some simply claimed the earth: 'I can cure cancer', boasted Rupert Wells throughout the American press at the turn of the century, 'At home, without pain, plaster or operation, and I tell you how, Free.' At around the same time, S.R. Chamlee advertised similarly in the American press:

> I WILL GIVE $1000 IF I FAIL TO CURE ANY CANCER OR TUMOR. I TREAT BEFORE IT POISONS DEEP GLANDS Without KNIFE or PAIN. No Pay until Cured. No X Ray or other swindle. An Island plant makes the cure. ABSOLUTE GUARANTEE.
>
> (Quoted in AMA, 1912: 33)

Others tried blitzkrieg advertising. James Eno, in the early nineteenth century, was the first practitioner to use whole-page advertisements in the press. These advertisements for his fruit-salts were extraordinary in their coverage and content, being completely taken up with allusions to national events, quotations from Plato, Browning, Thackeray, Pope and others, and homespun poems ('What nobler aim can Man attain Than conquest over human pain?'). 'Professor' Thomas Holloway, who marketed cure-all pills in Victorian England, was spending £20,000 a year on advertising by the mid-nineteenth century. He was the first world-wide advertiser of medical products. His name appeared on hoardings in London; it was to be found in newspapers of China, India and Peru; it even appeared on the Great Pyramid in Egypt.

The success of mass-advertised nostrums and a frankly commercial approach to healing raises interesting questions. It is likely that some patients chose such proprietary remedies because of their anonymity and impersonality, particularly in the case of embarrassing disorders like sexually-transmitted diseases. Others may have felt that patent medicines gave better value-for-money than the vaguer advice about 'regimen' they were likely to get from their regular practitioner. As commodity relations grew more important in a commercial, industrial society, there was perhaps a new 'magic' in having something tangible to take, swallow, rub in or apply: it gratified the need in an exchange economy to have something tangible for your money.

Some quack advertisers tried to win confidence through publishing testimonials of reports of cures. Thus the *Daily Advertiser* of 10 June 1736 puffed Joshua Ward:

> We hear that by the Queen's appointment, Joshua Ward, Esq; and eight or ten persons, who in extraordinary Cases have receiv'd great benefit by taking his remedies, attended at the Court at Kensington on monday night last, and his patients were examin'd before her Majesty by three eminent surgeons, several persons of quality being present, when her Majesty was graciously pleas'd to order money to be distributed amongst the patients, and congratulated Mr Ward on his great success.

Others appealed to fear, as did the American the Rev. Dr Bartholomew, who marketed an Expectorant Syrup. In 1860, under the ominous heading 'Last Day', Bartholomew noted that consumption 'usually sweeps into the grave, hundreds of the young, the old, the fair, the lovely and the gay', and he asked the reader 'Have you a cough? – Do not neglect it: – Thousands have a premature death from the want of a little attention to the common cold.'

There were scores of ways of drawing attention. Some developed special packaging, distinctively shaped and coloured bottles, trade marks and brand names (helped, especially in nineteenth-century America, by generous patenting laws). 'No cure, no pay' was a common line.

Quack doctors piloted gimmicks. Some boasted they took their own pills.

> To show its safety, sovereignty and efficacy, either when in health or sickness, Mr Patence constantly *takes his own pills* to preserve his own health, and gives them to children even in the mouth, in all cases.
>
> (Quoted in Thompson, 1928: 344)

The sugar-coated pill was pioneered. These pills, easier to swallow than the horrid concoctions prepared by physicians, were introduced into America in the eighteenth century by patent medicine makers like Zadoc Porter and C.V. Clickener. 'Heretofore,' Clickener advertised, 'medicine in almost all its forms was nearly as disgusting as it was beneficial'. But 'CLICKENER'S PURGATIVE PILLS, being completely enveloped with a COATING OF PURE WHITE SUGAR (which is as distinct from the internal ingredients as a nut shell from the kernel) HAVE NO TASTE OF MEDICINE.' And of course there was the special offer. Dr William Brodum in the 1790s, advertised 5 guinea bottles of his medicines. Smaller quantities came in three sizes, priced at £1 2s 0d, 11/6 and 5/5 a bottle. Brodum advertised the £1 2s 0d bottle as containing 'Five times the quantity as the 5/5 one'. (One could save 5/1 by taking the remedy in this way). Similarly Patence, who said of his 'Universal Medicine',

> if they do not answer the end proposed, I will return the Money. The real *worth of a box is Ten Guineas* but for the benefit of all, with proper directions, it is sold for three shillings; with personal advice, ten and sixpence.
>
> (*Morning Chronicle*, 1776, quoted in Thompson, 1928: 343)

Thus, orthodox medicine had forced quacks to 'sell themselves'. The development of capitalist institutions encouraged the big sell. Quacks took their opportunities.

FRINGE THERAPEUTICS

Behind the advertising stunts, however, there had to be some source of medical authority, to prove why the fringe medicine was superior to the orthodox. Some quacks nailed their colours to the mast of nature cures and folk wisdom. Many people loathed the polypharmacy of orthodox medicine. Such 'blunderbuss' treatment was both hit and miss and expensive. The treatments seemed artificial, and produced harsh and unpleasant effects, such as violent vomitings and purges. John Wesley summed up these objections thus:

> They consist of too many Ingredients. This Common Method of compounding and decompounding medicines can never be reconciled with Common Sense. Experience shows that One Thing will cure most disorders at least as well as twenty put together. Then why do you add the other nineteen? Only to swell the Apothecary's bill: Nay, possibly on purpose to prolong the Distemper, that the Doctor and he may divide the Spoil.
>
> (Wesley, 1747: xv–xvi)

Against polypharmacy, quacks often recommended old folk cures. Magical charms and amulets were marketed, such as the Famous Anodyne Necklace, whose beads speeded up teething in children. The beads were claimed to be made of the bones of St Hugh, who reputedly had cured children's diseases. When he dipped his finger in holy water and rubbed it nine times over a child's gums, the tooth came through. The Anodyne Necklace was marketed around 1720 by the Chamberlen family of male midwives and probably made them more money than their forceps. Herbal remedies were often recommended, such as 'ANGELICA. For the treatment of coughs, colds and pleurisy'; or 'BROOM. Used in the treatment of kidney and bladder infections'. Herbal cures seemed to have been signposted by God as specifics for particular diseases because of their 'signatures'. Thus the seventeenth-century English botanist William Cole wrote,

> *Wall-nuts* have the perfect Signature of the Head: The outer husk or green Covering, represent the *Pericranium*, or outward skin of the skull, whereon the hair groweth, and therefore salt made of those husks or barks, are exceeding good for wounds in the head.

Patriotic nineteenth-century American herbalists took the view that God would provide: the American countryside was bound to contain within it all herbs sufficient for the cure of the American sick.

The appeal to natural and simple cures could be made in more subtle forms. One was homeopathy, developed by Samuel Hahnemann in late eighteenth-century Germany. Hahnemann put forward the principle of treating like with like (for instance, that fever-inducing drugs should be used to fight fever), and also believed in the efficacy of very small doses of especially pure drugs, partly because in his view orthodox medicine habitually overdosed.

Alternative practitioners who advocated nature and folk remedies did not on the whole expect to make their fortunes through selling patent medicines. Their greater chance of fame came through publications. From Culpeper's *Herbal* onwards there was a growing spate of books expounding the principles of simple and self-medication to the reading public, such as A. Hume's *Every woman her own physician* (1776), or W. Smith's *A sure guide in sickness and health* (1776). They advocated direct and cheap remedies, as for example these from John Wesley's *Primitive Physick*:

A STUBBORN CHOLICK

Drink largely of *Camomile Tea*.
Or, of Decoction of *24 Mallow Leaves*:
Or, take from forty to an hundred Drops of
Anniss-seed Oil in a little Sugar.
Or, half a Dram of *Maetick*, mixt with the
Yolk of a new-laid Egg twice a day.
Or, apply outwardly, a Bag of *Hot Oats*.

(Wesley, 1747: 41)

This genre also emphasized what might grandly be called 'preventative medicine': the elementary principles of hygiene and healthy living, all stress diet and moderation; exercise and cleanliness figure prominently in works such as William Buchan's *Domestic Medicine* (1769). Other fringe medical publications were books of sexual advice. One of the most lastingly popular works was *Aristotle's Master Piece*. This compendium of sexual folklore first appeared in English in 1684 and was frequently re-edited. It discussed subjects such as the determination of the sex of children, the effect of the mother's imagination on the embryonic child, the birth of monsters, and the reasons for infertility. Perhaps the most famous English writer of sexual advice was James Graham, who in 1783 published his *Lecture on the Generation, Increase, and Improvement of the Human Species! Interspersed with Precepts for the Preservation and Exaltation of personal Beauty and Loveliness; And for prolonging Human life, Healthily and Happily, To the very longest possible Period of Human Existence! . . . And . . . closed with a glowing, brilliant, and supremely delightful Description of the Structure, and most irresistibly Genial Influences of the Celebrated Celestial Bed!!!*

The appeal to nature wisdom was especially pronounced in the case of women healers. Until late in the nineteenth century all women healers were by definition quacks, because they were excluded by law from medical education and the medical corporations. The rural areas of Europe were studded with 'wise' and 'cunning' women (in French, '*magies*'), quasi-witches who had for centuries dispensed medicines as well as brewing potions to put spells on one's enemies, or make a damsel fall in love or the butter set. But some healers attained wider fame, and their medical credentials generally rested on access to higher Natural or Supernatural powers. In Cheshire in the 1740s an old woman called Bridget Bostock cured 'the blind, the deaf, the lame of all sorts, the rheumatic, King's Evil, hysteric fits, falling fits, shortness of breath, dropsy, palsy, leprosy, cancers, and, in short, almost everything, except the French disease, which she will not meddle with'. What she did was to pray over her patients and stroke them with her spittle (it had to contain no trace of food, so that she had to treat all her patients before she broke her fast). In Catholic countries it was women who were usually the instrument in miracle cures. The healing grotto of Lourdes was discovered after a peasant girl, Bernadette Soubirous had a vision of the Blessed Virgin Mary, who announced to her 'I am the Immaculate Conception'. Similarly, the mushroom growth of spiritualism, especially in the United States in the nineteenth century, was led by women faith-healers. It was a woman, Mary Baker Eddy, who set in motion the biggest faith-healing movement, Christian Science.

Other elements of fringe medicine have created credibility by claiming to be more scientifically up-to-date than orthodox medicine. It has never been difficult to levy the charge of antediluvian traditionalism against the medical establishment, since tradition and precedent were its very watch-words; Galenolatry was still powerful in the seventeenth century, and the eighteenth century produced a neo-Hippocratic revival. In the sixteenth and seventeenth century 'empirics' such as Paracelsus could side with the Moderns in the 'Ancients versus Moderns' debate, and advocate new chemical specifics for disease, such as mercury as a treatment for syphilis. A couple of centuries later it was the scientifically and politically radical but medically marginal Thomas Beddoes who, with the young Humphry Davy, recommended nitrous oxide as a cure for consumption at his Pneu-matic Institute near Bristol. Advocates of magnetic cures, such as Mesmer with his special tubs, or Perkins with his tractors, were always able to claim to be ahead of the medical establishment in the van of scientific progress.

Fringe claims to be in the van of science seemed specially attractive when the cure was embodied in mechanical apparatus. For example, the Constant Current Cure Company of New York was advertising an electrical generator in the 1870s which would cure all diseases:

Headaches, Neuralgia, Rheumatism, Pains in the Back, Loins, Limbs, and Kidneys, Extreme Weariness, Nervousness, Insipient Consumption, Piles, Malarial Aches and Pains, Indigestion, Sleeplessness, Debility, Exhaustion, Liver Complaint, and all other *diseases requiring the peculiar stimulation afforded by a constant electric current.* This gentle stimulation of the affected part induces nutrition in that region, and gives nature the aid required to set all of the repairing agencies actively at work.

This powerful yet simple and compact generator develops a con-tinuous, mild electric current, capable of passing entirely through the human body, affecting every organ, nerve, and tissue, producing marked curative effects.

The current, although so subtle and permeating, is not perceptible to the senses, yet it will operate a galvanometer through a resistance of 5,000 ohms, equal to a telegraph line over 300 miles long.

This truly scientific instrument is indorsed by physicians and elec-tricians, and *will cure when all other things fail.*

Fringe practitioners were commonly able to carve out new domains for themselves with the aid of new medical technology. This was made the easier because orthodox medicine decried specialization, and also had tradi-tionally neglected certain fields of sickness as *infra dig* or uninteresting.

Obstetrics had been left to women. The rise of the male midwife from the seventeenth century was closely linked with the development of forceps. Eye, throat and ear specialists emerged in the nineteenth century alongside instruments such as the ophthalmoscope and the laryngoscope.

I have so far discussed two types of authority successfully appropriated by quacks: what a Weberian would call 'traditional authority' (the appeal to nature and folk wisdom), and 'rational authority' (the appeal to science). More potent than either of these, and lying behind both of them, has been the appeal to the third of Weber's categories: charismatic authority. Many fringe practitioners have exerted an appeal superior to orthodox medicine because they have seemingly combined the qualities of leader, priest, prophet and redeemer. Orthodox medicine quite early became – to use Weberian terminology again – routine and bureaucratic. It had opened up a professional chasm between physician and patient, which was to widen with the growth of clinics and sophisticated technology. With its heavy somaticism, and its materialistic and mechanistic emphasis upon drug therapy, it increasingly treated the disease and not the patient. From Sydenham onwards – one might almost say from Hippocrates – emphasis was on the observation of symptoms rather than the causal explanation of sickness.

Yet patients asked more than this from medicine. People discontent with their own lives, their families, their career, their prospects, their lovelife, disconsolate, frustrated, feeling a failure – such people, often ill, depressed, distressed, needed explanations for their misfortunes and new meaning for their lives. They might seek explanation and solace in religion, in politics, in philosophies of moral self-improvement (yet orthodox churches had themselves become bureaucratic, stressing virtue and ritual rather than conversation and redemption).

The promise of the quack was to transcend these bounds. Not to be just to relieve bodily pain or save souls – the dichotomized and dislocated parts of the human whole; but to heal. The quack might be a healer of the whole person, making sickness and its cure take on meaning as purposeful processes, as rites of passage to a better life.

Quacks have always been able to play upon the huge pool of melancholy experience and high hopes in any population. People whose psychophysical experiences have been a disappointment: the short, the fat, the inarticulate, the impotent, the aging, the unsuccessful, the shy, the spotty. They have been prepared boldly to identify such people as failures; to predict worse horrors to come (astrology was important here), and to attribute blame to the patient himself: self-abuse, self-neglect, self-indulgence have brought on the condition. Illness, pain, debility, are the wages of evil or ignorance. Such guilt-inducing ploys have obviously been particularly effective in the case of patients already ashamed by their own course of life: those suffering from venereal diseases, from alcoholism, obesity, psychological disorders.

But – like the traditional hell-fire preacher – quacks have also held out the hope of salvation by therapy (frequently, and significantly, only with the cooperation of the sick themselves).

This bold vision of the healer's art frequently involves the claim that the practitioner possesses special quasi-priestly, thaumaturgical powers. He may be in contact with the spirit world, or be able to tap vital fluids of the universe or exorcize distempers. Orthodox, somatic medicine distanced itself from spiritual healing. The Anglican Church rejected it in the eighteenth century as 'enthusiastic'. After Queen Anne, English monarchs disclaimed thaumaturgical powers. Where the orthodox feared to tread, quacks moved in.

Part of the quack's charisma has lain in his claim to reveal, grasp and utilize a hidden cosmology, and even, magus-like, to manipulate the occult powers of the cosmos. This alternative natural philosophy frequently has been animist, vitalist, voluntarist and monistic, proclaiming the ultimate unity of all existence and its suffusion with spiritual forces. At one with nature, the healer perceived the health-giving properties of nature's basic, elemental forces. As Jung's psychoanalysis would predict, healers have emphasized the symbolic associations of these archetypes. Thus water has had enormous cachet as a cure amongst marginal medical men. Water has great resonance as an agent of cleanliness and purification. It is the matrix of life and the symbol of baptism and rebirth. It has been deployed in fringe therapies in multitudes of ways: pure fresh water drunken as a cure for disease; cold water baths in hydrotherapy; sea water taken internally and externally; and most commonly healing mineral springs. Within temperance and teetotal movements, water became almost a medicine.

Other alternative therapies claimed to be able to tap and manipulate different elemental forces. Particularly from the eighteenth century onwards, practitioners sought to harness the immaterial, ethereal, electrical and magnetic powers of the cosmos – powers seen as the key to life, or the principle of vitality. They were thought especially valuable for treating nervous complaints such as epilepsy and melancholy, because both were in some sense 'spiritual'. John Wesley's diary contains numerous instances of his using electrical therapy.

Electro-magnetism was also recommended for sexual debility (because 'animal magnetism' contained the principle of attraction). James Graham, for instance, developed the 'Celestial Bed' for curing impotence and infertility, which worked through the forces of electrical fire:

The chief principle of my Celestial Bed is produced by artificial lodestones. About 15 cwt. of compound magnets are continually pouring forth in an everflowing circle. . . . The super-celestial dome of the bed, which contains the odoriferous, balmy and ethereal spices, odours and essences, which is the grand reservoir of those reviving invigorating influences which are exhaled by the breath of the music and by the exhilarating force of electrical fire, is covered on the other side with brilliant panes of looking-glass.

(Graham, 1780: 151)

Graham presented himself as a high priest at what he called his Temple of Health, with young female priestesses who assisted 'at the display of the Celestial Meteors, and of that sacred Vital Fire over which she watches, and whose application in the cure of diseases, she daily has the honour of directing'.

Others have recommended the curative powers of Mother Earth. Mud baths in particular have enjoyed vogues from time to time. James Graham was, once again, one of their strong advocates. Presumably re-emerging from a mud bath had overtones of resurrection.

Air, too, has had its advocates. The virtues of fresh air were stressed more and more in family health manuals. Thomas Beddoes hoped to develop inhalation of gases as a cure for consumption, in 1799 opening his Pneumatic Institute for Relieving Disease by Medical Arts at Clifton near Bristol. The basis of pneumatic medicine (as it was called) was the idea that ordinary air, consisting of nitrogen and oxygen, was chemically changed in the lungs and became almost pure oxygen.

Not least the virtues of 'ozone' were trumpeted. Ozone generators went on sale in late nineteenth-century America. 'Ozone' said one advertisement,

is nature's disinfectant, and no disease can exist in a malignant form where it is in the atmosphere. It renders sewer gases harmless. In Diphtheria and Scarlatina its effects are wonderful. In Intermittent, Marsh, or Malarial fevers it is of inestimable value, and Fever and Ague cannot exist where there is Ozone. It removes the offensiveness of the sick chamber, filling it with fresh and pleasant odours.

We supply Ozone Generators in two sizes; prices $3 50 and $5 00. Orders by post promptly attended to. Send for pamphlet. HEKTOGRAPH CO., 22 and 24 Church St., New York.

The most universal and holistic of these archetypical cures was the appeal to the panacea. Back in the sixteenth and seventeenth centuries panaceas were still being offered within the intellectual tradition of an alchemy which confidently looked forward to finding – or claimed to have found – the elixir of life. As alchemy became discredited, this intellectual frame-work was eroded, but still medicines were advertised under the name of 'elixir', with all its associations, supposedly curing an enormous variety of diseases, or more generally ensuring good health and long life, and retarding ageing.

The appeal of the quack has been to restore, not just to relieve physical pain, but to make born a new person; not just that, but to put the world to rights. Quacks have often been moral, social and political reformers, wanting to cure ills on the widest possible scale. Pain and suffering have been seen as the consequences of the radical misorganization of society and false values. Society needed to be cured along with the individual. A good instance is Lydia Pinkham in nineteenth-century America. Brought up in a Quaker household, Lydia Pinkham early embraced most liberal and humanitarian causes, including abolitionism and temperance. She dabbled with spiritualism and phrenology, currency reform and vegetarianism. She launched her own fringe medicine, the Vegetable Compound, quite expressly as part of her own feminist platform. She believed that male doctors were insensitive to female complaints. 'Only a woman understands a woman's ills' she believed. Testimonials from women using the Compound confirmed the popularity of a medicine attached to a cause. 'I had doctored with the physicians of this town for three years,' read one such letter, 'and grew worse instead of better.'

As should be evident from the above, it would be historically simplistic to try to pin alternative healers down to narrowly defined role models. Forced to the margins, they necessarily had to develop a range of acts and tactics. A man such as James Graham excelled in exuding charisma; but he was clearly also a fine entrepreneur with a grasp of consumer psychology that would match Josiah Wedgwood and an understanding of the commercial networks of a modernizing society. Successful fringe healers have to be all things to all people.

CONCLUSION

I have been trying to address the question: why has quackery had such huge appeal, so lastingly? I have stressed two kinds of answers. First, by being forced out of the élite world of medicine, fringe medicine was actually dumped in the most fertile seedbed of all: the capitalist market-place in the age of rampant capitalism (an arena which in most respects orthodox medicine chose to deny to itself). Second, fringe medicine could move into an area of human experience and need largely abandoned by orthodox medicine and orthodox religion. Orthodox medicine increasingly treated just the body, in ways unintelligible to the patient. Orthodox religion made promises for an immaterial soul in the hereafter. By contrast marginal medicine actually appealed to a sense of the whole person – the unity of mental and physical experience – and sometimes also to two other unities: the oneness of the person with the world, and the cooperation of patient and doctor. Quacks often spoke in languages which people understood.

Problems attend any overall assessment of the historical appeal of quack doctors. Because they were professionally and legally marginalized (and occasionally even criminalized) they have left less solid documentation than the physicians who rose to become presidents of royal colleges. The evidence – for example, grossly inflated handbills – is hard to interpret: massive advertising might be regarded as a mark of success, or it might be seen as a sign of desperation. As with pop groups today, there was a rapid turn-over in quacks. Eye-catching publicity was of the essence, but fashions never last.

It is clear, however, that regular practitioners felt obliged to take the threats posed by quacks seriously. In many cases, regulars attempted to hound and harry alternative practitioners. The strength of official regulation certainly curbed the spread of fringe medicine in France and Germany. In free-trade Britain and the United States, regulars often took a leaf out of the quacks' book. Asked by a medical student for some advice about how to set up successfully in practice, the doyen of late-eighteenth-century American physicians, Benjamin Rush, replied: study the quacks. His contemporary, Dr Erasmus Darwin, a Midlands practitioner and grandfather of Charles, gave precisely the same advice to his physician son. Evidently it was widely believed that fringe practitioners possessed better customer psychology, greater commercial flair, and a more winning manner with patients than their orthodox brethren.

The response of the public (then and now) bears this out. Particularly in the era of pre-scientific medicine, disease was king and regular medicine a weak reed. The rational recourse for a sick person was to try anything and everything. As we know from the letters and diaries of the sick in earlier centuries, they frequently consulted with a gaggle of doctors all at once. And sometimes they found in the alternative healer qualities their regular doctor lacked: gentler methods, more natural therapies, more winning or persuasive ways, or beliefs that harmonized with their religious outlooks. The fringe healer may thus have possessed placebo power to a greater degree than the regulars. Orthodox medicine has long pooh-poohed the placebo effect, while acknowledging its existence, seeing it as little better than magic. Today, as sensitivity is perhaps growing to the psychosomatic dimensions of sickness, some strands of regular medicine are beginning to take the placebo effect more seriously. The consequence might be moves to the reconciliation of orthodox and fringe healing.

REFERENCES AND FURTHER READING

Cooter, R. (ed.) (1988) *Studies in the History of Alternative Medicine*, London: Macmillan.

Coward, R. (1989) *The Whole Truth: The Myth of Alternative Health*, London: Faber & Faber.

Fielding, H. (1755) *Journal of a Voyage to Lisbon*, London: A. Miller.

Graham, J. (1780) *A Sketch, or Short Description of Dr Graham's Medical Apparatus*, London: Almon.

Holbrook, S.H. (1959) *The Golden Age of Quackery*, New York: Macmillan.

Inglis, B. (1979) *Natural Medicine*, London: Collins.

Jameson, E. (1961) *The Natural History of Quackery*, London: Michael Joseph.

Porter, D. and Porter, R. (1989) *Patient's Progress: Doctors and Doctoring in Eighteenth-Century England*, Cambridge: Polity Press.

Porter, R. (1989) *Health for Sale: Quackery in England 1650–1850*, Manchester: Manchester University Press.

Porter, R. and Porter, D. (1988) *In Sickness and in Health: The British Experience 1650–1850*, London: Fourth Estate.

Thompson, C.J.S. (1928) *The Quacks of Old London*, London: Brentano's.

Watts, G. (1922) *Pleasing the Patient*, London: Faber.

Wesley, J. (1747) *Primitive Physick*, London.

Young, J.H. (1961) *The Toadstool Millionaires: A Social History of Patent Medicines in America before Federal Regulation*, Princeton, NJ: Princeton University Press.

Young, J.H. (1967) *The Medical Messiahs: A Social History of Health Quackery in Twentieth-Century America*, Princeton, NJ: Princeton University Press.

4   The equation of responsibility

Complementary practitioners and their patients

Ursula Sharma

This chapter addresses the question of whether the healer–patient relationship in complementary therapy is radically different from that which obtains in orthodox medical practice. One very widespread opinion is that not only is this difference great, but it may be the very source of complementary medicine's current popularity. For example, Rosemary Taylor (1984) has argued that it is the deterioration in the quality of the 'medical encounter' consequent upon the overly technological approach to healing and (in Britain) upon overstretched resources which has caused many to turn to the more personal approach offered by most forms of complementary therapy.

This is a view which is often endorsed by the medical profession itself. While the famous (or infamous?) report on alternative therapies published by the British Medical Association in 1986 failed to approve alternative therapies, it did admit that while time and compassion were a part of good orthodox medical practice, many orthodox doctors worked in conditions where they could not give much of either to the individual patient. Alternative practitioners, it was argued, were often in a better position to do so, making them attractive to many patients even if their remedies were scientifically unproven (BMA, 1986: 74). Murray and Shepherd, writing in the *Journal of the Royal College of General Practitioners*, also suggest that patients of complementary practitioners appreciate the

> consolatory benefits of a lengthy consultation with a sympathetic therapist

and that

> Whereas formerly doctors were able to provide comfort and support to patients but not always much in the way of effective therapy, the general practitioner now offers a more comprehensive service, but with a consequent diminution in the time available for lengthy discussion.
> (Murray and Shepherd, 1988: 512–13)

What is the evidence that the relationships between healer and patient in complementary and orthodox medicine are fundamentally different? If there is such a difference, is it due to divergent philosophies of healing, different conditions of work, different demands made by the patients, or different attitudes and values on the part of the healers?

ORTHODOX MEDICINE

The type of relationship which a healer entertains with a patient and the quality of the communication between them will depend very much on personality and temperament, and this goes for both orthodox and complementary healing. However, this relationship will also be informed by ideological concerns about what the relationship ought *ideally* to be like (implicit or explicit in the healer's training) and shaped by the institutional context within which the practitioner is *actually* obliged to work.

Orthodox medicine is a broad church – possibly it encompasses as much diversity in terms of moral and clinical outlook as the various complementary therapies taken together. However, an important ideal of very general persuasion in the orthodox medical profession is the concept of clinical autonomy (Tolliday, 1978). If the doctor (and no one else) has, by virtue of his or her training, the necessary knowledge to treat the patient, then no other person or agency ought to have the right to dictate to the doctor what kind of therapeutic decisions should be made. In this respect the doctor is responsible to the patient alone. Yet in practice most doctors in Britain do not work as freelance or self-employed professionals, accountable only to patients and to their fellow professionals conceived as a kind of self-regulating brotherhood. They work in the context of medical bureaucracies and their responsibilities to their employers and to other doctors cannot be ignored (BMA, 1988a: 54). Professional texts which deal with the duties and responsibilities of doctors acknowledge the plural nature of much medical responsibility and attempt to clarify how the twin principles of clinical autonomy and of the primacy of the patient's interests may be seen in relation to the doctor's undoubted responsibility to his or her employer, whether the NHS or some other agency (BMA, 1988a, 1988b).

However, while individual doctors are subject to management of various kinds, they normally participate in a well-structured system of delegation or referral of very wide scope, which enables the patient to benefit from a far wider range of medical expertise than any one doctor might command. The general practitioner, the source of primary health care, may delegate 'up' (to a hospital consultant) or 'down' to a member of one of the paramedical professions (e.g. a chiropodist or physiotherapist). The General Medical Council has recently ruled that doctors may refer patients to complementary practitioners provided that they are satisfied of their competence to provide the necessary treatment. However, the doctor is conceived as retaining overall responsibility for the patient's treatment:

> a doctor who delegates treatment or other procedures must be satisfied that the person to whom they are delegated is competent to carry them out. It is also important that the doctor should retain ultimate responsibility for the management of his patients because only the doctor has received the necessary training to undertake this responsibility.
>
> (GMC, 1987, quoted in BMA, 1988a: 15)

Medical sociologists and anthropologists have noted that in practice this model disempowers the patient. The patient has a right to choose a doctor but his or her right to exercise choice in respect of treatment does not figure in this equation of responsibility, or at any rate not as it is set out in the kind of texts I have referred to. Individual practitioners sometimes do refer the choice of treatment to the patient when they are satisfied that there is more than one beneficial option, and many will seek to take into account the personal and social circumstances which might make one therapeutic option preferable to another for the patient concerned (e.g. Lefever, 1990), but they do this in spite of rather than because of the institutional constraints of their situation. It is not surprising, therefore, that the patients we encounter in medical discourse are 'compliant' or 'non-compliant', 'co-operative' or 'uncooperative', 'consent' or 'refuse', are 'put' into hospital. Not only medical conditions but patients themselves are 'managed'. This vocabulary implies that they can never be equal participants in choices or decisions, for this organization of responsibility rests on the principle that therapeutics involve the deployment of a specific medical expertise which the patient does not have. Numerous studies have traced the way in which medical power is established and exercised, some concentrating on the institutional setting in which doctors as a professional group are able to exercise control and exact deference (e.g. Freidson, 1970; also Margaret Stacey's contribution to this volume). Others have looked at the way in which control and deference are achieved in actual doctor–patient encounters (e.g. Bloor, 1976).

This equation of responsibility has not gone unquestioned by doctors themselves. There are certainly those (especially in the field of primary health care) who can envisage an equation of responsibility where the patient (expert on his or her own capacities, feelings, condition) collaborates with the doctor (expert in scientific medicine) (Tuckett *et al.*, 1985). Patrick Pietroni and other 'holistic' practitioners have pursued the idea of a form of practice where the doctor recognizes the patient's own knowledge and priorities. This kind of questioning can surface more easily in those areas of medical practice where there is not simply one self-evidently preferable type of treatment to which the doctor must direct the patient or else be open to charges of negligence. In some forms of cancer, for instance, there may be no such clear-cut imperatives, only a number of possible treatments, each of which may produce some benefits but each of which will also have drawbacks in terms of side-effects, discomfort, etc. The patient's insight into his or her own temperament and circumstances in such cases may be recognized as a resource the physician should draw upon.

Where patients seek an equal and collaborative relationship which is not endorsed by the individual physician, they expose a contradiction which lies at the heart of modern medical practice – that between an ethic which declares that the patient's needs and interests must always be the physician's priority, and the professional insistence that practice is based on a specific form of knowledge (increasingly technical and scientific) which can only be acquired through training, and is therefore inaccessible to the patient (see Lyng, 1990: 158ff for a discussion of this contradiction). Patients who seek collaboration in areas where orthodox medical opinion does not admit of uncertainty as to what is the best treatment or with a physician who prefers a hierarchical relationship are liable to be regarded as problematic. The fact that it is possible to write an article with the title 'The Informed Patient – Burden or Ally?' (Blair, 1985) is symptomatic of this contradiction.

Patients who use complementary medicine but conceal the fact from their general practitioner on the grounds that they do not wish to damage their relationship with a doctor whom they respect and whose services they value are seeking to avoid a confrontation with this contradiction (Sharma, 1992: 55ff). In choosing complementary medicine they have exercised their own discretion about what kind of expertise might be relevant to their condition, but they do not wish to risk incurring the displeasure of that doyen of orthodox medical knowledge who has the power to act as gate-keeper to important diagnostic and therapeutic services within the NHS which they may wish to use in future.

COMPLEMENTARY MEDICINE

Now it is time to turn to complementary medicine and consider whether we find different constructions of what I have called the 'equation of responsibility' in this field of therapeutic endeavour. First of all I consider the ideologies which practitioners refer to and the ways in which these ideologies might be expected to affect their practice; second, I examine the effect of the institutional context within which complementary practitioners practice; finally I discuss the kinds of pressure which might be expected to proceed from patient demands and expectations.

I refer to various sources of information but draw extensively on two small-scale studies which I carried out between 1986 and 1990. The study of patients involved extensive semi-structured interviews with thirty people who had used some form of complementary medicine in the past six months. The second study comprised semi-structured interviews with thirty-four practitioners of complementary medicine who were working in or in the vicinity of an industrial town. Both were carried out in Midlands localities. (For fuller accounts of these studies, see Sharma, 1992.)

Complementary medicine and holistic ideologies

The category 'complementary medicine' is difficult to delimit and comprises a very wide range of therapeutic activities and interventions. We must be careful, therefore, about undue generalization. However, most claim to be holistic in some sense. At the most general level these claims are made by organizations which represent the therapies and seek to communicate the benefits of their methods to the general public (e.g. professional organizations) and by practitioners who write about their system of healing for the general public. I found that all except one of the practitioners in my study re-iterated such claims, and most mentioned it spontaneously when describing what they tried to do for patients in practice.

Holism comes in many forms and degrees and as a therapeutic ideal is by no means confined to the complementary therapies, having particular appeal among GPs and among nurses. In its weakest form, holism means treating the patient's symptoms not in isolation but as part of a total health profile, taking into account a wide range of information about the patient and his or her circumstances, preferences, state of mind, etc. One leaflet on homoeopathy, for example, claims that

> homoeopathy recognises that all symptoms of ill health are expressions of disharmony within the whole person and that it is the patient who needs treatment, not the disease.
>
> (Leaflet published in 1988 by the Society of Homoeopaths)

Another states that

> Osteopaths who belong to the British Naturopathic and Osteopathic Association approach the patient as an individual and have a traditionally holistic attitude to the treatment of disease. In other words, even though two patients may have the same symptoms, the osteopath may treat them differently because the cause of the symptoms may be different in each case.
>
> (Leaflet issued by the British Naturopathic and Osteopathic Association)

Many of the practitioners who took part in Peter Davies's 1984 study of complementary therapists commented that some of the questions in the questionnaire (on whether they gave nutritional advice) were difficult to answer because, for example,

Acupuncture does not treat the symptom but the patient.

(Davies, 1984: 29)

There is a general emphasis on the very individual nature of holistic treatment. An experienced homoeopath describes her practice thus:

I always ask myself 'How is this person different from another with this particular complaint?' The homoeopath individualizes the prescription to fit the patient – rather like a tailored suit. Imagine that the body is a jigsaw. Prescribing on one symptom alone is like seeing only a small part of the jigsaw; it does not give you enough information to work out what the whole picture is.

(Castro, 1990: 13)

One obvious implication of this approach for the relationship between the practitioner and the patient must be that the therapist is going to need much more information from the patient, information which only the patient can provide. Some complementary therapies involve special expert methods of scanning the body (practitioners of traditional Chinese acupuncture monitor pulses on different parts of the body, chiropractors and osteopaths use various forms of palpation, some herbalists use iridology, which involves the examination of enlarged photographs of the iris). But to the extent that the therapist also needs to know about the patient's circumstances and feelings, much detailed information must be elicited which only the patient can deliver, on which the patient alone is the 'expert'.

This, of course may be no more than what a good orthodox practitioner aspires to do, and some orthodox doctors have pointed out rather resentfully that the complementary therapies can hardly be said to have a monopoly of this kind of holism (Williams, 1989: 60). However this may be, there is certainly evidence that complementary practitioners spend much longer on the process of examination and history-taking than orthodox GPs; the average length of first consultation in my sample of practitioners was one hour, and for subsequent consultations a little under three-quarters of an hour. These times are somewhat higher than those which Davies's study of practitioners yielded, the average time for first consultation among his sample being thirty to forty-five minutes and for subsequent consultations sixteen to thirty minutes with, however, much variation according to therapy (Davies, 1984: 20).

If consultations are lengthy this need not be solely because the practitioner needs time to gather information from the patient; many complementary practitioners whom I interviewed saw it as an important part of their work to explain treatment and offer general advice on the prevention of further problems to the individual patient:

> I normally try to explain to all my patients exactly what is going on in layman's terms as far as possible, because I think people really want to know what is going on anyway, they like to try and understand what is going on. I explain why certain things help, why certain exercises are going to help, and then once it makes sense to them I think it makes them want to do it more.
>
> (Osteopath)

Some took an even more robust view of their educational responsibilities:

> That is why I talk about teaching all the time because it is about convincing people, about educating them and then about motivating and keeping them motivated . . . giving them every piece of information they could want and a lot more they haven't asked for.
>
> (Herbalist/iridologist)

There is, however, a stronger form of holism which involves more than simply treating the symptoms which the patient presents in the context of a total profile of that person's life and circumstances. This form of holism involves the explicit encouragement of the patient to take on more responsibility for his or her own health. The objective here is not simply the elimination of the problem which has caused the patient to consult in the first place through the mobilization of the body's healing resources, but also a progress in self-understanding and self-responsibility.

> I just see myself as a catalyst of people getting to know for themselves what is needed. Everyone leaves here with a programme [of dietary advice]. But it is their responsibility when they leave here and their choice as to how much they actually do with that. . . . what I try to do is teach them what they need to do to make their life work, not to create dependency.
>
> (Reflexologist/herbalist)

> . . . another thing I try to do is help the individual to understand that they are the only person that can heal themselves and that what they are doing when they come to someone like myself is finding systems or methodologies which they can heal themselves with, and that takes away the possibility of dependency . . . they are being re-educated into healthy harmonized individuals.
>
> (Healer/shiatzu)

This generally goes with the tenet that the patient's problems are likely to be more complex than the presenting symptoms suggest. Illness is likely to have more than one cause, and the healer's responsibility is to dig into these possibly unconscious causes. This idea is not exclusive to complementary medicine (see Siegel, 1990, for an 'orthodox' surgeon's version of what I call 'strong' holism) though it is unlikely that many GPs will have the time or resources to pursue multiple causation in any depth.

> Sometimes they come with one problem and you know there's another problem, but it's a sort of problem you hope they will talk about.
>
> (Acupuncturist)

> Some people come here and they have a chronic stress problem, but they come for reflexology and they say reflexology is what I want, nothing more. . . . I say, fine, so they go on to [the reflexology] and when they start to relax they start to say, I have got too much weight and I don't sleep very well and everything else.
>
> (Reflexologist)

Where the problems are much deeper and unknown, or not acknowledged by the patient, the therapist has to tease them out:

> I have a really good feel about people, I can usually tell if I am getting some resistance or there is a grey area that they don't want to go into. . . . I always like to create a settled environment and space and give people time, and it is amazing what comes out then.
>
> (Reflexologist)

> [the length of treatment] depends on me and it depends on how many consultations we need to go through before the patient can face the cause of the problem, because sometimes we can't deal with an issue directly, they have got to deal with another issue before they will deal with that one.
>
> (Hypnotherapist)

Some practitioners made the point that, so far as they were concerned, it was the patient who set the agenda for the consultation initially and that they would try to ascertain what the patient him/herself wanted from treatment – alleviation of symptoms? Cure of a specific condition? General improvement of well-being and preventive care? However, if the causes of ill-health are deep-seated, then the consultation is likely to offer scope for redefinitions of the agenda:

> What I do tends to open people up and as they open up they tell me things and I try to help them. All pain, in my mind, is blocked energy and it manifests as physical disease and you work at it from that level.

You work on it from the ground upwards and you get the physical stuff sorted out. Once the physical stuff begins to sort out you discover that there is emotional garbage there, you work on that a little bit and you may find that there are patterns of behaviour associated with it, and you find that maybe the whole alignment of their life is wrong.

(Osteopath)

Some commentators have seen holists' emphasis on the cultivation of self-responsibility as positively dangerous. For one thing it may justify and even nourish a neo-conservative advocacy of cut-backs in publicly provided health care; if individuals are capable of taking responsibility for their own health, then why should they make excessive demands on the state (Wikler, 1989: 144)? For another thing, it may open the way to moralistic victim-blaming; if individuals are responsible for their own health, may it not be their own fault if they are ill (Coward, 1989: 93)? I have some sympathy with these criticisms, for they are not trivial. The personal *right* to take responsibility for one's own health is all too easily elided with the civic *duty* to take this responsibility (with the certainty of censure and the possibility of penalties for those who fail in this respect). However, neo-conservative thinking about health service provision will probably have its day irrespective of any contribution from holistic practitioners, whether orthodox or complementary. The question we need to address here is: does this kind of approach to therapeutics ultimately *empower* patients (because they end up more able to take charge of their own health and with a better insight into the roots of their own problems)? Or does it *disempower* patients (because whatever therapists may say about not creating dependencies, patients cannot do without the healer's insight and assistance through what may be quite an uncomfortable process of exploring the profundity of their own motivation, their 'need to be sick')? In short, does this not suggest a very directive role for the therapist in the short term even if the long-term goal is the empowerment of the patient, and even if holistic healers exercise control in a very different way from the orthodox physician? As one therapist said,

I fit in with the patient, I am fluid, I am what the patient wants me to be. But I am in the driving seat even though they do not know it.

(Homoeopath)

This is a difficult question to answer without a careful investigation of what complementary therapists of the 'strong holism' tendency actually do, as opposed to the ways in which they decribe their ideals and therapeutic objectives, and this is something which is not particularly well documented as yet. As indicated in some of the interview extracts above, the therapist may well encounter resistance from the patient. Several practitioners spoke of the problem of dealing with patients whose notions of what constituted treatment were quite narrow. Several interviewees admitted to sometimes encountering problems in persuading patients to undertake regimes of diet, exercise, etc. which they were convinced would be beneficial but which the patient regarded as contrary to local common-sense notions about what makes you better and what makes you ill (see below), never mind regimes which involve the opening up of unsconscious motivation. One suspects that patients eventually match themselves to therapists whose approaches they find acceptable and that some patients simply fail to return to a therapist whose notions about therapy are fundamentally at odds with what they are prepared to accept, or who propose a radical revision of the sense of self when symptomatic relief is what the patient insists upon.

What about the issue of re-education – does this not imply a fairly directive role for the practitioner? In this respect do complementary practitioners adhere to a very different model of the distribution of responsibility from that which governs orthodox practice? After all, orthodox physicians will usually tell the patient as much about their condition as they feel the patient ought to know, and will explain what the patient should do to prevent a recurrence of symptoms. On the other hand, health education of a broader kind is regarded as a special activity, separate from therapy and entrusted to a different set of professionals. If it is the expertise of the doctor which – as we saw in the case of the orthodox equation – legitimates medical control over therapy and the doctor's acceptance of final responsibility for the case, then does not the complementary therapist's preparedness to share knowledge also open up the possibility of shared power – a genuinely more equal and collaborative relationship?

> Basically I think it's important that you explain what you're doing. There is a danger otherwise that you become the next élite, with all the power, and that's what the orthodox medical profession often has done, and some of the other professions. . . . There would be little point if someone came in with raised shoulders that were stiff and I just gave a medical diagnosis. There's a reason they are holding their shoulders up, emotional protectiveness or whatever, and I need to explain that to them. If they choose to do nothing with that knowledge, that's fine and I will have the prudence to leave well alone, but there are all sorts of ways in which you can re-educate people.
>
> (Masseur)

It is important to point out that practitioners such as this one did not see themselves in the business of teaching their patients how to become masseurs, how to diagnose homoeopathically or to perform manipulation.

Rather they claimed to educate the patient about his or her *specific* problems, to offer what information that *particular* patient needed or could make use of. Whilst in the case just quoted the masseur's client becomes more expert on his or her own problems, the masseur remains the professional expert on massage.

Perhaps to pose the question simply in terms of whether the relationship between practitioner and patient is more or less hierarchical is to miss the point. And, assuming that power is the issue at all, maybe it is misleading to speak as though the balance of control between practitioner and patient were some kind of zero-sum game in which empowerment of the one must weaken the other (even if that is the way in which orthodox medical discourse often approaches the therapeutic encounter). If these healers are doing what they say they would like to do, then they are leading the patient through a process of self-awareness in which the balance of control between patient and healer shifts over time. The ideal which they hold to is one in which patients initially seek some form of help which they cannot provide for themselves, draw on the healer's expertise, then gradually become more independent and self-reliant with respect to their health and well-being. Holism in the strongest form is more akin to psychoanalysis in that it sees the interaction between healer and healed as an ongoing process rather than a static relationship (see Susan Budd's contribution to this volume). Even in its weaker form it often involves much scope for the revision of agendas and redefinitions of the task in hand by both the patient and the practitioner.

Complementary medicine: the institutional context

I argued earlier that most orthodox doctors operate within a bureaucratic context and that this has an inevitable effect on the relationship between healer and patient, being conducive to a hierarchical definition of relationships. Individual physicians may have their own characteristic ways of handling patients and may hold different views on how much information patients ought to be given, but the pressures of the institutional context will do much to determine the range of behaviours which are either permissible or productive both for doctors and for patients.

Some complementary practitioners work within the NHS and are presumably exposed to the same constraints, no doubt one of the factors which makes some other complementary practitioners chary about integration into the NHS (see Cant and Calnan, 1991: 53; Sharma, 1992: 211). At present, however, the majority work as freelance self-employed professionals who receive fees from patients in proportion to the number of consultations. My own study suggested that a fairly high proportion of complementary practitioners may have other sources of income (e.g. from lecturing on their therapy or training others to practise it) but these will usually be on a contract basis. A characteristic of some of the therapists was a positive distaste for working within a large organization, a desire to have control over one's own working conditions even at the expense of security. This was particularly true of some therapists who had formerly worked in the NHS (usually as nurses) and were appreciative of the greater therapeutic autonomy they felt they enjoyed as independent practitioners (Sharma, 1992: 131). Cant and Calnan record a similar taste for freedom to practise. As one of their interviewees (a naturopath) said:

> I don't want to be clumped with GPs. Everything has a place but we should not all be clumped together. . . . I wouldn't like to work in a clinic. I like to be in charge.
>
> (Cant and Calnan, 1991: 53)

However, many practitioners work in a group practice of some kind. Davies (1984: 17) found that exactly half of the respondents in his sample of practitioners worked with one or more other therapists, not necessarily from the same discipline (9 per cent worked with conventional doctors). In my own much smaller sample only a third of the practitioners worked alongside others, none with orthodox doctors. The kinds of partnership and cooperation which complementary therapists engage in are quite variable. At one end of the range we have the loose pairing of complementary therapists who work alongside each other in a simple literal sense, sharing premises and perhaps the services of a receptionist. At the other end of the range we find the integrated clinic including both orthodox and non-orthodox healers where the patient comes to the clinic rather than to the practitioner and is directed to whichever services or treatments are considered appropriate for his or her particular problems, and where there may be case conferences at which the individual patient's progress is discussed by a group of collaborating practitioners. Genuinely integrated clinics seem to be unusual at present though they may become more common in future, but there are an increasing number of holistic health centres in which some degree of collaboration over cases and/or mutual referral obtains among the member practitioners.

Complementary therapists, therefore, tend to work in settings characterized by a non-hierarchical ethos and minimum of direct control from either superiors or equals. Thus they appear to have the clinical autonomy and freedom from managerial interference which orthodox doctors hold as an ideal, but without the control exercised by professional colleagues which doctors also hold to be the main safeguard against poor standards of practice. Indeed this apparent conjunction of liberty and non-accountability may explain the particularly hostile attitude which some orthodox doctors entertain towards complementary practitioners.

However, this institutional detachment carries its own constraints, especially lack of access to certain kinds of resource. At the most basic level, for instance, a chiropractor in my sample complained that whilst she could often make better diagnoses and plans for treatment with patients' X-rays before her, she had no means of obtaining these under the NHS, thereby making the treatment more expensive for the patient. Information about the patient's past treatment is another resource to which the GP has access, in the form of the patient's medical notes, denied to the complementary practitioner. Some therapists (mainly homoeopaths and osteopaths) saw it as very relevant to their plan of treatment to know what drugs or other treatments their patients had been prescribed in the past. Indeed many homoeopaths will wish to know about treatments, operations and inoculations carried out in early childhood, which not all adult patients are likely to remember accurately or in detail. Recent moves to make it easier for patients to have access to their medical records may help resolve this problem, but there is still no institutionalized channel for the communication of such information between GPs and independent complementary practitioners. Usually, therefore, the therapist has to rely on what patients can manage to recall.

A greater problem, I suspect, is the lack of referral resources. An orthodox GP can refer patients with serious or complex problems to a hospital consultant, indeed one of the very important functions of the GP is to act as gatekeeper to these specialized services. Hospital consultants themselves may refer patients to other services and there are formal systems of communication among all these different persons and agencies. If this occasionally means that patients whose problems are difficult to diagnose or regarded as psychosomatic in origin get passed around from one medical specialist to another, it also means that individual doctors can feel that there are other resources to call upon for a patient when their own clinical knowledge or experience is inadequate to the case.

What resources can complementary practitioners draw upon when they feel that they can do no more for a patient who is still far from well? Some practitioners take quite careful steps to avoid getting into the situation where their resources to help the patient 'run out' by turning away patients whose condition they do not think they can substantially improve.

> I don't treat any cancer whatsoever. I wouldn't take on multiple sclerosis either, it is not curable. Some of the obvious degenerative nervous conditions I wouldn't take on either. I am very selective about

who I would take on in that sense. We are talking about the chronic type patient who is going to spend a lot of money and not get anywhere.

(Acupuncturist)

An osteopath was careful to discourage patients who came expecting more than she knew she could achieve for them:

they always look for the sensational, the patient who crawls in and is able to run out, that is what they are looking to be, and they come expecting miracles. . . . It's sad really.

Another osteopath described how he effectively screened patients when he first took their history:

If you have any suspicion [that the patient has cancer] you have got to look at them in great depth and make your decision what to do. If I suspect that someone has cancer what I would do is, I am afraid, get rid!

In my sample the practitioners who did this tended to be fairly confident and experienced.They had built up local, even national, reputations which were not going to suffer if they frankly admitted their inadequacy in the face of a few grave or incurable conditions.

Many practitioners could think of instances where they had advised a patient to consult his or her GP about symptoms which they suspected presaged a cancer or some other serious condition, even if they did not conduct such systematic 'screening'. However, most people who consult a complementary practitioner have already consulted an orthodox doctor for the condition that troubles them (see, e.g., Moore *et al.*, 1985: 28; Thomas *et al.*, 1991: 209). If a patient has run through the gamut of orthodox treatments and come to complementary medicine as a last resort, it will be a very tough-minded practitioner who will find it easy to deny some little hope, and why should a well-trained healer not have faith in his or her own discipline to do some good in such cases, even if a complete cure cannot be found?

On the other hand, the lone therapist who takes the risk of accepting a really difficult case has few further resources to offer the patient in the event of total therapeutic failure. A practice which is becoming common in some therapies (notably homoeopathy) is for recently qualified practitioners to come together regularly in a 'supervision' group where they can discuss difficult cases with a more experienced colleague. There are also various kinds of support group where therapists who work in isolation can simply exchange experiences and provide mutual encouragement. Occasionally such support groups bring together practitioners of different therapies. Most of the practitioners whom I interviewed had some links with others in the area, and about half could be described as 'active networkers', that is, they participated in informal or semi-formal communication or meetings with other practitioners on a fairly regular basis, some being prepared to refer patients on to such practitioners and to receive referrals from them (see Sharma, 1992: 152). One hypnotherapist described her practice thus:

> If I don't feel that someone is making enough progress then I will say have you tried this or have you tried that? You get some people who for instance really have medical conditions which are better treated by a homoeopath and I refer them to Dr X, because I have heard very good reports of her. I also know a Bach Flower Remedies practitioner who, again, if anyone needs that kind of treatment, I can send them to him.

An osteopath told me:

> If I don't think I am getting there as quickly as I ought to I will try and think of somewhere to refer the patient that might just help them more. Another osteopath or an acupuncturist.

One or two interviewees even quizzed me tentatively about practitioners of disciplines other than their own in the area, presumably with a view to augmenting their referral resources. This curiosity, however, was tempered with the much more frequently expressed fear of associating oneself with therapies which the interviewee did not regard as genuine or reputable, not to mention individual practitioners whose competence could not be assured. Some practitioners preferred to battle on with the sole responsibility of a difficult case rather than encourage the patient to consult others. As one acupuncturist said:

> I can only guarantee the standard of my own work, and not that of anyone else.

I am discussing therapeutic failure as a limiting situation which will test the patient–practitioner relationship and reveal the extent of the resources upon which the practitioner can call, and not because there is any particular evidence from my studies that it is a common problem for healers. Therapeutic failure is in any case defined by the patient in the end, and most studies of patients' perceptions of complementary medicine, both in Britain and in other countries, indicate fairly high levels of satisfaction (see, e.g., Fulder, 1989: 35; Parker and Tupling, 1976: 375). Talking to patients, one also realizes that for some who are chronically or even terminally ill, what the therapist has done is to help them come to terms with their illness rather than cure it. One interviewee in the study of patients was an advanced cancer patient who described her experiences with a spiritual healer. She told me that while her symptoms continued and she did not expect any great improvement, the healer had taught her how to cope with the pain and disability which she suffered. Others described benefits which would not conform to an orthodox doctor's notion of a complete clinical cure, but which were clearly regarded as well worth the fee paid in the patient's judgement (see Sharma, 1992: 84).

Some orthodox doctors have seen this kind of case as demonstrating that complementary therapy has no real clinical effects; it may cheer patients up and make them more hopeful but this does not entitle it to claim therapeutic efficacy. This is not the place to resolve the question of what constitutes clinical efficacy in complementary medicine, how it should be tested and by what criteria it should be judged – issues which have been reviewed much more widely since the Bristol Cancer Help Centre controversy exploded in 1990. However, it is worth noting that according to the holistic view of therapeutics, at least according to what I have called the 'stronger' version of holism, the claim that complementary medicine (or any other kind of healing) acts on the mind rather than the body is in itself no argument against it; the comfort and sustaining of the patient and the cultivation of optimistic fortitude is an important aspect of compassionate therapeutics, disposing the physical 'part' of the (whole) person to mend. If we take this view (and obviously some patients do), then whilst lone therapists may 'run out' of resources in terms of options for referral or further intervention, their compassionate attention may constitute a resource which is extremely valuable and (in theory at least) need never 'run out'.

One hypnotherapist described a long-standing patient for whom she felt she could do little more until that patient's appalling domestic circumstances changed. However she continued to see her when the patient rang her up because,

> She has nobody else and I tend to feel I am doing her some good. Some people would say that if you see someone for that long you have a case of dependency, Freudian transference, that what you are doing is making them dependent on you. In certain circumstances that is quite true, but everyone needs a friend and if I can be a friend to someone and see them blossom a little under that friendship then I am perfectly willing to do that.

What I have tried to demonstrate in this section is that in some important respects the medical encounter in complementary medicine is bound to be different from that which obtains in orthodox medicine, and for reasons which are only partly to do with therapeutic ideologies and much to do with the institutional environment. Complementary therapists, unlike orthodox GPs, do not act as gatekeepers to further resources which can be offered to or withheld from the patient, and therefore they lack a potential source of control over the patient (even assuming that they might wish to exercise such control). A person registered with a GP may consult infrequently or not at all, but can be said to have some kind of long-term relationship with that doctor (recognized by the state), however tenuous and devoid of affective content. The relationship with a complementary practitioner may be quite intense while treatment is in progress, but it is also potentially brittle; the patient who decides that a particular practitioner is doing nothing for the illness need never consult again and the relationship simply ceases to exist. Orthodox doctors' integration into a bureaucratized system of health care delivery also gives them access to a wide range of resources and skills which can be deployed to help a patient whose case is difficult to treat.

As we have seen, therapists do not claim to experience this as a major problem and can devise means of coping with this situation far short of giving up the independence and autonomy which they value. It does mean, however, that the balance of the relationship between the patient and practitioner rests on a different kind of fulcrum and involves a different configuration of responsibility.

CONSUMERISM AND THE EQUATION OF RESPONSIBILITY

Most complementary medicine is sold on the market. Now, markets beget consumers – the patient is customer as well as client. Does not the customer–provider relationship denote a very different equation of responsibility from the professional hierarchy which I depicted at the start of this paper? Customers should be able to call the shots, although we all know that in restricted markets they may find it difficult to do so. We would imagine in a very fragmented market like that for complementary health care, where providers are mainly individuals or small groups with relatively little collective social or economic power, that the customer would be king, being free to leave the therapist for another the moment the treatment appears (by whatever criteria the patient chooses to employ) not to merit the money spent on it. In the consumer model of health care the patients take responsibility for their own health by exercising their judgement about the kind of care relevant to their conditions in the first place. In short, the self-responsibility which is the aim of the 'strong' model of holism is the starting point for the market model.

Some have queried whether it is useful to apply the concept of consumerism to health care. Margaret Stacey has argued that in some important respects it is not. In the NHS the patient is the *object* of a work process, unequal in power to the person who controls this process (Stacey, 1976). British Rail passengers who shiver as they wait for a train which will arrive late, if at all, will appreciate the irony of applying a market model to a monopoly service, and will deride the loudspeaker announcement which appeals to them as 'customers'. We should also be suspicious of discourse which appeals to a consumer model when it is the doctor who is envisaged as making consumer choices rather than the patient.

Certainly much confusion results from talking about choice and consumerism when the person who exercises the choice is not the person who 'consumes' the service, that is, the person who is ill. But could we not argue that it is quite legitimate to talk about consumerism in the kind of private health care market in which most complementary medical services are sold? And that the implications of the consumer–provider relationship for the equation of responsibility are considerable? Furthermore, is it not the case that the term consumerism can be used to denote a certain attitude of mind, a demanding approach to the product, whether the latter is offered on a free or a monopolistic market?

Some patients certainly seem to behave in a 'consumerist' manner in relation to health care in general, sifting and comparing information about the conditions from which they suffer and about the various known treatments, including complementary ones. Some of the interviewees in my study of patients confessed to having no special commitment to any particular form of medicine, but choosing whichever form of therapy seemed best for the illness or condition in question.

A characteristic example was a woman who suffered from chronic back pain, also low energy (depression?). She had been diagnosed as having cancer in the past and had a mastectomy;

> I went [to a chiropractor] off my own bat. But I was going oftener and oftener, and I seemed to get better for a while but I had a lot of personal problems which were contributing to the tension, stress and overwork. So I tried acupuncture and it seemed to help. . . . Through the acupuncturist's receptionist [who was his sister] I got to know about a herbalist and I still see him for constipation and bowel troubles. I take homoeopathic remedies for some things, arnica for bruises and pains.

The interviewees who manifested this kind of exuberant eclecticism were not the majority (ten of a sample of thirty). A further fourteen used one particular form of therapy consistently for one or more problems, and the rest could be described as being only at the stage of trying out complementary medicine to see what it could do for a particular problem rather than seeing it as a regular feature of their choices in health care. However, it is quite likely that this approach to personal health care will spread, especially if complementary therapy becomes more widely available under private health insurance schemes.

The fact that complementary therapists offer their services on a market basis to people who are increasingly taking a consumerist attitude to health care presumably means that sometimes they find themselves in a poor position to realize their commitments to heal their patients since the latter may abandon them at any time if they do not like the therapy which is offered. This, of course, may be true of orthodox medicine as well where complementary medicine is an affordable alternative. No wonder orthodox doctors are anxious about the possibility of large numbers of patients either abandoning orthodox medicine, or (which could be more difficult for them to deal with, given their particular notions about how therapeutic responsibility should be disposed) using orthodox and complementary medicine either simultaneously or serially. In this situation doctors cannot be sure what outcomes are the result of their own treatments and what may be the result of patients' experiments with other regimes. Worse still, the doctor may be blamed for some other therapist's failures.

> If a general practitioner regards the use of unorthodox treatment outside the NHS as potentially harmful, must he or she continue to accept clinical responsibility? What, for example, is the responsible course of action for the general practitioner who finds that a child is suffering as a result of unorthodox treatment selected by the parents without medical consultations?
>
> (Murray and Shepherd, 1988: 513)

Once there are multiple health care options, and once it is the patient who exercises the choice, the implications for the balance of responsibility between practitioner and patient are considerable.

But what of Taylor's argument, which I cited at the beginning of this chapter, that people turn to complementary medicine precisely because they perceive the practitioner as treating them with more consideration and dignity? Might not the quality of the healing bond be one of the very aspects of complementary medicine which attracts the punters? If that were true, then, taking the point of view of the therapist for the moment, the less hierarchical relationship which the complementary therapist offers can be seen (positively) as a market asset which attracts the new client rather than (negatively) as a source of vulnerability for the practitioner.

Survey data from a number of countries suggest that people consult in the first place because they have a particular condition (usually chronic but not life-threatening) which orthodox medicine has not cured to their satisfaction, rather than any ideological commitment to methods of either treatment or communication in complementary medicine (Fulder, 1989: 44; James *et al.*, 1983: 386; Thomas *et al.*, 1991: 210). Dissatisfaction with orthodox medicine is chiefly related to its treatment of particular kinds of illness, and only secondarily to aspects of the patient–practitioner relationship. This kind of data, however, may be a product of the way in which subjects have been interrogated in surveys. Those studies which invite patients to make explicit comparisons between orthodox and non-orthodox health care professionals often reveal considerable sensitivity to the quality of the complementary therapist's mode of communication. The Dutch study *What is Better?*, for instance, showed that users of complementary medicine were more likely to respond negatively to certain statements about the kind of relationship they had with their GP than were a control group of patients of orthodox consultants. The differences were not enormous but they enable us to say that people who used non-orthodox therapists were somewhat more critical of the orthodox medical encounter than patients of consultants, though it does not entitle us to conclude that this dissatisfaction was the cause of their resort to complementary medicine (Ooijendijk *et al.*, 1981).

When we ask patients about their experiences some do perceive a difference in the quality of the healing relationship in complementary medicine. As one of my interviewees described experiences with a herbalist:

> She treated me as an equal in intelligence and she convinced me that my problems were to do with the whole of my body. She took time to find out what was wrong, she explained everything to me. She even told me what my temperament was and helped me to come to terms with it.

CONCLUSION

At this point I find that I reach the limit of what I am prepared to argue about the patient–practitioner relationship in complementary medicine in general. To go further I would have to examine the characteristic ideologies and procedures in each of an ever increasing panoply of treatments. Even generalizing to the extent that I have done here could be dangerous, lest it be forgotten that within the particular professional communities that complementary medicine comprises there are certainly many local and personal variations, just as there are in orthodox medicine. What I have tried to show is that in most forms of complementary medicine found in Britain today there exist both therapeutic ideologies and institutional structures which at the very least make possible, and in the strongest case positively encourage, a relationship between practitioner and patient in which the latter can be a very active partner in treatment, much more active than most orthodox doctors would envisage or desire. In such a case the term 'patient' perhaps requires revision; sick people 'suffer' their sickness, but are not 'passive' in their suffering.

Such a case is not always realized of course. What transpires in the complementary therapist's consulting room need not be so very different from what transpires in the GP's surgery. The patient is interrogated and examined and a remedy is dispensed. But to the extent that the complementary practitioner usually operates quite independently of the state's interest in the bodies and health of its citizens there is always the potential for a very radical difference. Most complementary practice does not (at present) participate in the panoptical surveillance of citizens envisaged by Foucault.

A practitioner whom I interviewed recently used a completely different 'optical' image to describe her practice (one familiar to psychoanalysts; see Susan Budd's contribution to this volume), seeing herself as a mirror who reflects back an image of the patient's life; to the extent that patients are enabled to see aspects of their selves and lives which were not clearly perceived before, they can make use of this self-knowledge to facilitate healing. According to this healer, it is the patient who heals him- or herself, the practitioner merely provides favourable conditions and resources for this process. If the widespread incorporation of complementary therapies into the NHS ever becomes an issue, then both patients and practitioners would need to balance the (to my mind undoubted) advantages of wider access against the disadvantage that the opportunity to develop a more flexible and interactive relationship between healer and healed than that which the present NHS context encourages would almost certainly lose out to the requirements of political and bureaucratic accountability.

REFERENCES

Blair, P. (1985) 'The Informed Patient: Burden or Ally?', *Modern Medicine*, November: 28–32.

Bloor, M. (1976) 'Professional Autonomy and Client Exclusion: A Study in ENT Clinics', in M. Wadsworth and D. Robinson (eds), *Studies in Everyday Medical Life*, London: Martin Robertson.

BMA (1986) *Alternative Therapy: Report of the Board of Science and Education*, London: BMA.

BMA (1988a) *Philosophy and Practice of Medical Ethics*, London: BMA.

BMA (1988b) *Rights and Responsibilities of Doctors*, London: BMA.

Cant, S. and Calnan, M. (1991) 'On the Margins of the Medical Marketplace? An Exploratory Study of Alternative Practitioners' Perceptions', *Sociology of Health and Illness*, 13(1): 39–57.

Castro, M. (1990) *The Complete Homoeopathy Handbook*, London: Macmillan.

Coward, R. (1989) *The Whole Truth: The Myth of Alternative Health*, London: Faber & Faber.

Davies, P. (1984) *Report on Trends in Complementary Medicine*, London: Institute for Complementary Medicine.

Freidson, E. (1970) *The Profession of Medicine*, New York: Dodd, Mead and Co.

Fulder, S. (1989) *The Handbook of Complementary Medicine* (rev. and updated edn), Sevenoaks: Coronet Books.

GMC (1987) *Professional Conduct and Discipline: Fitness to Practice*, London: GMC.

James, R., Fox, M. and Taheri, G. (1983) 'Who Goes to a Natural Therapist? Why?', *Australian Family Physician*, 12(5): 383–6.

Lefever, R. (1990) 'Decision-Making', in B. Devlin, D. Freeman, I. Hanham, J. Le Fanu, R. Lefever and B. Mantell (eds), *Medical Care: Is it a Consumer Good?*, London: IEU Health and Welfare Unit.

Lyng, S. (1990) *Holistic Health and Biomedical Medicine: A Countersystem Analysis*, New York: State University of New York Press.

Moore, J., Phipps, K. and Marcer, D. (1985) 'Why Do People Seek Treatment by Alternative Medicine?', *British Medical Journal*, 290: 28–9.

Murray, J. and Shepherd, S. (1988) 'Alternative or Additional Medicine? A New Dilemma for the Doctor', *Journal of the Royal College of General Practitioners*, 38: 511–14.

Ooijendijk, W., Mackenbach, J. and Limberger, H. (1981) *What is Better?*, Netherlands Institute of Preventive Medicine and the Technical Industrial Organization, London: translated and published by the Threshold Foundation.

Parker, G. and Tupling, H. (1976) 'The Chiropractic Patient: Psycho-social Aspects', *Medical Journal of Australia*, 2(10): 373–9.

Sharma, U. (1992) *Complementary Medicine Today: Practitioners and Patients*, London and New York: Tavistock/Routledge.

Siegel, B. (1990) *Peace, Love and Healing*, London: Rider.

Stacey, M. (1976) 'The Health Service Consumer: A Sociological Misconception', in M. Stacey (ed.), 'The Sociology of the NHS', *Sociological Review Monograph*, 22: 194–200.

Taylor, R.C.R. (1984) 'Alternative Medicine and the Medical Encounter in Britain and the United States', in J. Warren Salmon (ed.), *Alternative Medicine: Popular and Policy Perspectives*, London: Tavistock.

Thomas, K., Carr, J., Westlake, I. and Williams, B. (1991) 'Use of Non-orthodox and Conventional Health Care in Great Britain', *British Medical Journal*, 302: 207–10.

Tolliday, H. (1978) 'Clinical Autonomy', in E. Jacques (ed.), *Health Services*, London: Heinemann.

Tuckett, D., Boulton, M., Olson, C. and Williams, A. (1985) *Meetings between Experts: An Approach to Sharing Ideas in Medical Consultations*, London: Tavistock.

Wikler, D. (1989) 'Holistic Medicine: Concepts of Personal Responsibility for Health', in D. Stalker and C. Glymour (eds), *Examining Holistic Medicine*, Buffalo, NY: Prometheus Books.

Williams, S. (1989) 'Holistic Nursing', in D. Stalker and C. Glymour (eds), *Examining Holistic Medicine*, Buffalo, NY: Prometheus Books.

Part II
Problems of regulation

5 Collective therapeutic responsibility
Lessons from the GMC

Margaret Stacey

For the purposes of this chapter I distinguish between individual therapeutic responsibility and collective therapeutic responsibility. My concern will be with the second, although that both influences and is influenced by the first. Individual therapeutic responsibility is exercised by the practitioner in the encounter with a client or patient. Collective therapeutic responsibility is expressed in the formal rules or advice promulgated by organizations of practitioners which guide or restrain individual practitioners in encounters with patients or clients. The purpose of such rules or guidance is to control the standards of practice and behaviour of members. When those formal rules or guidance have statutory backing the constraints experienced by the practitioner are tighter because the sanctions which the professional body may exercise have legal authority.

The General Medical Council (GMC), which regulates the British medical profession, is often seen as the archetypical controlling body and is not infrequently used as a model for the regulation of other professions. The General Dental Council, for example, has marked similarities with the GMC. A more recent example is the General Osteopathic Council, enacted in 1993, whose structure and functions closely resemble those of the GMC.

Historically, the establishment of the GMC and the advancement of the profession were closely connected. From this a belief seems to have arisen that state registration confers professional prestige. This, I suggest, is a mistaken assumption. Nor do I believe that certain occupations have inherent in them characteristics or traits which mark them off as 'professions' (see also Johnson, 1972). Rather, in my view professions are simply occupations which have made claims to professional status supported by particular organizational arrangements. Such occupations are differentiated from each other by how far their claims have been recognized.

Occupations which make claims to professional status tend to share certain characteristics. One is the control, based on educational criteria, of entry to an occupational association, and, in the case of state registration, control extends so that those not on the register may not claim the registered title. The qualifications demanded require a more or less extended period of education and training. A register of those admitted is kept. When the state recognizes such occupations, those on the register may be accorded further privileges, as, for example, the monopoly granted to registered medical practitioners in state employment, such as the armed forces, and in the NHS. State recognition does not, however, automatically confer the same status and power upon all professions who achieve it. The differences between the privileges and status accorded to doctors, dentists, nurses and the professions supplementary to medicine demonstrate this.

The pros and cons of state recognition will be discussed more fully later in this chapter. A major part of the argument will rest upon the differences among the wide array of non-official modalities, avoiding a simple dichotomous division between orthodox (or official) and complementary medicine (see the Introduction to this volume; also Saks, 1992a: 2–4, and Sharma 1992a: 5–7, for other terminological uses, and the discussion in Stacey, 1988: chap. 11). Official medicine, which originated in allopathy, I shall refer to as 'biomedicine' because of its basis in biological science. Furthermore, although I am aware that biomedical practitioners are not altogether happy with it, I shall use 'healer' and 'healing' as technical terms applying to all those occupations whose practitioners seek to cure or reduce illness, pain or suffering.

Whether it is wise for all health care occupations seeking to become professions to take the General Medical Council, with which the state has for many years had an exclusive accord, as the model of collective therapeutic responsibility to which they should aspire must be open to question. Furthermore, if at all, when or for whom might this be an appropriate aspiration? The question also arises as to how the state should view the plurality. To answer these questions one first needs to understand the arrangements on which the GMC is based and how they have come about.

THE GMC: HISTORICAL BACKGROUND

Professional self-regulation and state registration

Since 1858, what is now biomedicine has been controlled by the GMC through a method of professional self-regulation supported by a statutory system of registration and the doctrine of clinical autonomy. According to the Merrison Inquiry, set up to investigate the medical profession, professional self-regulation can be seen

> as a contract between public and profession, by which the public go to
> the profession for medical treatment because the profession has made

sure it will provide satisfactory treatment. Such a contract has the characteristic of all freely made contracts – mutual advantage.

(Merrison Report, 1975: para. 4)

The circumstances in which biomedicine gained such a special relationship with the state over against other modalities were historically specific. The new biomedical practitioners in the late eighteenth and early nineteenth century made alliances with the rising bourgeoisie who were to become of increasing importance in British government (Peterson, 1978; Waddington, 1984). When later the state greatly expanded its activities, biomedical practitioners were the ones the state employed. The GMC was at the crux of this mutually beneficial alliance between biomedicine and the state. Indeed during the 1930s, as Larkin (1992a: 6, and see also Larkin, 1992b: 115–18) has put it, the Council was so closely involved with government it was in reality 'treated as another department of state'. This may well have been the case throughout: we lack evidence.

Privilege moves towards monopoly

From 1858 onwards the register maintained by the Council enabled the public to recognize qualified from unqualified practitioners, as the Act put it (quoted Merrison Report, 1975: para. 2). Only those on the register of the qualified could call themselves 'registered medical practitioners'. Other practitioners, the so-called 'unqualified', were not made illegal, but the state reserved certain tasks for the registered, such as recording 'births, fitness, sickness and death' (Larkin, 1992a: 3). By 'qualified' was meant qualified in ways which were acceptable to the Council. Slowly a standard-ized education was achieved.

As biomedicine became more powerful, restrictions increased. The 1939 Cancer Act, for example, forbade 'anyone but a registered medical practitioner from treating, or offering to treat, cancer, by advertisement or any other means', a provision inserted by the British Medical Association (BMA). Bright's disease, cataract, diabetes, epilepsy or fits, glaucoma, locomotor ataxy, paralysis and tuberculosis were added in the 1941 Pharmacy and Medicines Act. The National Health Insurance (1911) and the NHS (1948) Acts restricted contracts and posts to registered medical practitioners. So members of the public who wish to receive treatment from therapists of any other modality have had to 'go private'. The increase in and resort to unregistered practitioners over the last ten to fifteen years is the more remarkable since, in the face of biomedical treatment free at the point of delivery (but paid for out of taxes), with few exceptions, patients of any other modality have to pay for the services they receive.

The historical view reveals a number of issues about the lessons to be learnt from the GMC: individual occupations being organized to train and to discipline their practitioners to ensure high standards of skill and care; freedom to practise, freedom from state restriction; the value of state patronage. The last gives a competitive advantage over other healing modes. Where the state is proactive in the health field the preferred modality has a great advantage over all others in terms of the resources available to it, financial, legal and social. Any retreat of the state from active involvement has the potential to leave more space for other modalities.

Dominating the division of labour

The terms under which nurses, midwives and the professions supplementary to medicine were registered, whereby they were subservient to biomedicine, show clearly that state registration of itself is not adequate to ensure an occupation a status such as that of biomedicine. On the contrary, biomedicine used its privileged position as the official state modality to establish a division of health labour in which it was dominant (Larkin, 1983; Stacey, 1988: chap. 6). Most, although not quite all, of those professions which were registered but subordinated were, initially at least, composed entirely or predominantly of women (Stacey, 1988: chap. 6; Witz, 1992).

Keeping the profession together

A united profession is needed for self-regulation to work. The great differences among allopaths partly explain why thirty years elapsed before Parliament passed an Act setting up the GMC (Waddington, 1984). The unity of the profession has been maintained by insisting on the essential equality of all registered medical practitioners one with another, whatever might be their specialism, practice circumstances and material status. Medical unity rests on this political philosophy, and its associated organization and actions, rather than on a common knowledge-base. This somewhat fictional unity is continually tested.

Maintaining legitimacy

Closely associated with maintaining unity and also in order for professional self-regulation to work, the Council (like the regulatory body of any occupation) has to maintain its legitimacy within the profession; it has to take the registered medical practitioners with it. In the late 1960s and early 1970s it nearly lost this legitimacy. Some senior as well as many junior doctors felt the leadership was out of touch with contemporary health care organization and medical practice and with the experiences of the practitioners of the day. A revolt was precipitated by Council's decision to institute an annual retention fee if doctors wished to keep their names on the register. When this turmoil threatened the proper running of the NHS the state finally stepped in and set up the Merrison Inquiry into the regulation of the profession which eventuated in the 1975 report quoted earlier (for a fuller account see Stacey, 1992a: chap. 4).

Around this time, with its future in doubt, the Council recorded its view that the 1858 Act

> was passed largely as a result of initiative within the profession, and the establishment of the Council was *desired as much for the protection of the duly qualified medical practitioner from the competition of unqualified practitioners as for the protection of the public*.
>
> (GMC Minutes CX, 1973: 179; my emphasis)

Research evidence suggests this statement, later published as a pamphlet, 'Constitution and Functions', is correct (Saks, 1992a; Waddington, 1984).

Protecting the public

The medical profession used its influence in the Department of Health and the Houses of Parliament to prevent the Merrison Committee from looking at the principle of professional self-regulation which underlies the constitution and functions of the GMC. State registration has worked to the advantage of biomedicine over against other healing modalities and other health care occupations. Until recently at least it served the state to the latter's satisfaction notwithstanding frequent disputes between the profession, or sections of it, and successive governments (see also Larkin, 1992a: 9).

Has it served the public well? This is, after all, the chief function of the GMC as it well knows, a statutory duty laid upon it. My research suggests that the medical profession gained rather more than the public out of the bargain.

THE MODERN GMC

My research on the Council

I joined the GMC as a lay member at about the time the Merrison Report was published. The focus of my research (Stacey, 1992a) – which I undertook a decade later – was on the tensions the Council experienced between maintaining the unity of the profession, on the one hand, and protecting the public, on the other.

As I got further into it, this research presented me with a conundrum:

The Council's members and leaders are people of high ethical standards who care about the delivery of a good health service, believe they are doing a good job and continually strive to do better. Yet they operate a system of regulation which neither ensures the continuing competence of practitioners, nor adequately disciplines the incompetent.

(Stacey, 1992b: 123)

I found that in practice the Council has tended to lean towards the protection of the profession rather than of the public.

A professionals' Act

The Council was reformed as a result of the Merrison Inquiry in ways which restored its legitimacy but also strengthened the professional bias. A main change made by the 1978 Medical Act, later consolidated into the 1983 Medical Act, was to give a majority on the Council to elected representatives (and thus increase the influence of the BMA) as opposed to persons nominated by the Queen in Privy Council (that means effectively by the health ministers) or appointed by the royal colleges and university medical schools. The size of the Council was more than doubled to ninety-three but the proportion of lay members actually declined. Seven out of ninety-three is roughly the same as three out of forty-six on the unreformed Council, but the six 'truly lay', if one may so call those with no health care qualification, amounted to a smaller proportion than previously (Stacey, 1992a: 84). Including the new arrangements for the registration of overseas doctors (see below: The 'Register'), this was a professionals' Act, designed to solve problems within the profession rather than improve the protection of the public.

The functions of the GMC

In 1973, in evidence to the Merrison Committee, the GMC, referring to the objective in the preamble to the 1858 Act that 'it is expedient that persons requiring medical aid should be enabled to distinguish qualified from unqualified practitioners', wrote:

the whole of the Council's functions flow from that original objective ... the general duty of the Council is to protect the public, in particular by keeping and publishing the Register of duly qualified doctors, by ensuring the educational standard of entry in the Register (and thus in the profession) is maintained, and by taking disciplinary action against registered doctors if it appears, by reason of their misconduct, that they may be unfit to remain on the Register.

(Quoted in the Merrison Report, 1975: para. 2)

My evidence for suggesting that the Council leans towards the profession rather than the public comes from examination of the three tasks of the GMC listed in the quotation above.

1 The register

The first function quoted, that of keeping and maintaining the register, gives the GMC power to control entry and maintain discipline. There are at present three principal and certain other subsidiary lists. The first three are the main register (or principal list), that is, those who have been granted full registration; the second is the list of those provisionally registered; the third, the list of those who have limited registration. There are, in addition, lists of those who have been granted temporary full registration; a list of fully and provisionally registered doctors who are currently working outside the United Kingdom; and, for EC purposes only, a list of doctors holding certain specialist qualifications. There is as yet no register of specialists, although specialist qualifications may now be included in the main register.

Those on the main register have gained qualifications approved of by the Council, that is, those granted by British medical schools and a (now small) number of overseas medical schools. Before being admitted to this register graduates serve a 'pre-registration' year during which they gain practical experience. For this purpose, after passing their examinations, graduates are put on the provisional register so that they may practise under supervision. Those qualified overseas have to demonstrate that they have gained equivalent experience before being admitted to full registration. Limited registration, which replaced temporary registration after the 1978 Act, is used for other doctors qualified overseas and is for only five years. To get on the limited register a doctor should have a hospital post and either have passed certain clinical and linguistic tests or be sponsored. Doctors may be admitted to full registration by transfer from the limited list, having fulfilled certain qualifications, the details of which need not concern us here. Furthermore, the Council is actively considering establishing one method only of limited registration, which would remove the special status of recognized medical schools and put all incomers on a similar footing. (For further details of the distinctive treatment of doctors from the new Commonwealth, see Anwar and Ali, 1987; Moss, 1992; D.J. Smith, 1980; Stacey, 1992a: chaps 10 and 12.)

2 *Education*

Educational standards, the second function mentioned, are the responsibility of the Education Committee, since the 1979 Act technically independent of the Council but in fact working closely with it. As does the Council in other matters, the Committee works by achieving and maintaining consensus, in this case of medical educators as much as of the profession as a whole. It does not itself educate, train or test aspiring practitioners. That is done by medical schools, which are well represented on the Education Committee. The medical schools and non-university licensing bodies set and mark the examinations which students must pass to get on the register. The GMC exercises a general educational oversight partly by offering guidance to universities as to what should be included in the medical curriculum and also by its responsibilities as to the standards, appropriateness and organization of the qualifying tests and examinations.

The GMC guidance on medical education is derived from consultations with the senior teachers in the medical schools and only published with their agreement. The freedom of the medical schools to experiment is always stressed. This approach means that the guidance will be reasonably well received, that schools have advance warning of any proposed changes; the guidance will possibly be acted on but is rarely radical. Some medical commentators (e.g. Horder *et al.*, 1984) have suggested that the GMC guidance is ahead of what is actually taught in medical schools.

Take the example of undergraduate medical education. Many agree that the undergraduate medical curriculum contains too much didactic teaching and is cluttered with factual data which rapidly become out of date. However, teachers are reluctant to curtail or drop traditional subjects and are resistant to whole-scale changes in teaching methods: hence the present unsatisfactory situation. The GMC acknowledges that medical education may in these ways be inappropriate as a preparation for the practice of modern biomedicine, which itself changes rapidly as new research evidence is made available or technical advances open new ways of treating old complaints. Furthermore, medical practice takes place in a constantly changing society. Practitioners need to be able to think for themselves when applying medical knowledge rather than acting on the basis of rote learning.

In the 1989 Annual Report the chairperson of the Education Committee admitted:

> The Medical Act 1978 sought to allow greater freedom in medical education than before. It paved the way for a liberation of the curriculum which the Education Committee went on to encourage in its 1980 Recommendations on Basic Medical Education. But the shackles have

not been loosened in any significant way. Ten years on, we have embarked on a further review, seeking to tackle the problems afresh.

(*GMC Annual Report for 1989*: 17)

This review was published in December 1993 as *Tomorrow's Doctors* and includes proposals for radical curriculum changes.

The GMC has powers to inspect the examination of medical students. However, for 'no clearly minuted reason' (Kilpatrick, 1985: 8), no inspections were made of the older universities after 1959 (Crisp, 1983: 32). The President, when asked in 1978 why only the recently founded universities were inspected, said the Council 'did not find it necessary' to visit old-established universities. However the physicians and surgeons, through their royal colleges, jogged the GMC out of this complacency in 1981. When the inspections were introduced great care was taken not to cause offence to the universities (Stacey, 1992a: 111).

Initially the GMC only had responsibility for basic medical education, the royal colleges retaining principal control of postgraduate education. As medicine has developed, post-basic training has become increasingly important, the absence of a specialist register more significant, the lack of coordination of all stages of medical education the more serious. The 1978 Act gave the GMC responsibility for coordination, but few teeth to ensure it. The royal colleges and other bodies are reluctant to yield power and government has become increasingly impatient. One of the problems with the cluttered basic education, in the view of some, is that topics are being taught in the undergraduate years that should properly be taught after graduation. These problems, which echo disputes which have been around in medicine since before the GMC was formed, have not yet been fully resolved.

In its statement about the functions of the GMC quoted above, the Council claimed that by controlling standards of entry to the profession it controlled the standards of the profession. However, the Council has no means of knowing whether the standards insisted on at first registration have been maintained by practitioners nor whether they have kept up with changes in disease conditions and the treatments available. The Council makes exhortations about the need for doctors to undergo continuing medical education, but there is no system of re-registration (or re-licensure) or other mode of ensuring that current standards of practitioners' knowledge and practice are adequate. There are doctors, including at least one who has been a Council member, who feel this is needed if the public is properly to be protected. Any such system would be expensive and not popular with the rank and file. Some of the royal colleges are, however, considering some form of re-accreditation. It remains unclear in what way the GMC currently ensures standards are maintained.

3 *Fitness to practise*

The third function of the GMC is to see that those on the register are competent to practise. The Council was designed not to be the apex of a complaints machinery, but rather to maintain the reputation of the profession. It is the one body which can withdraw a doctor's right to practise. Its procedures are separate and serve a different purpose from the NHS complaints procedures; those relate only to doctors employed by or in contract with the NHS. Apart from the law, the GMC is the only body by whom doctors in private practice may be disciplined.

The Council has no inspectorate. Information reaches it about doctors convicted in the courts (all such convictions are or should be reported to the GMC by the Home Office); complaints come from officials of public bodies and from individual members of the public suggesting that a doctor may be unfit to practise. When such complaints are received they are sifted by the office, under standing orders from the President, as to whether they properly come under the jurisdiction of the Council. If they do, they are then seen by a preliminary screener who will consider whether the complaint may possibly be sufficiently serious to call registration into question. Formerly it was the President himself who did this; now he (the President has up to now always been a man) appoints preliminary screeners who act for him. Since 1990 these have included a layperson who sees all cases after the medical screeners have been through them and before the next step is finally decided.

Since the 1978 Act, an initial task of the screeners is to decide whether the problem may lie with the doctor's health (most usually alcohol or drug addiction); if that seems to be so, the matter is handled as a clinical problem by the preliminary screener for health. This person invites the doctor to undergo a medical examination and as long as the doctor concurs with this proposal and with any treatment and other advice (about practising at all or under supervision, for example) which may be offered, the case is treated in a strictly clinical manner. Only if the respondent doctor refuses to undergo medical examination or to conform to the treatment advised does the matter come to the formal Health Committee. This committee has powers of suspension for one year (renewable if necessary) and of putting conditions on the practice a doctor may undertake.

If, on the other hand, it seems that the doctor complained of may be 'bad' rather than 'mad' (or otherwise sick), the conduct procedures are invoked. Doctors referred to the conduct procedures have been convicted in the courts or are alleged to have behaved in a way which raises a question of serious professional misconduct. The preliminary screener for conduct first reviews the allegations: if she or he (the first woman screener has recently been appointed) decides there may be a case to answer but that further information should be sought, this is arranged.

The screener refers the potentially serious cases to a Preliminary Proceedings Committee which examines the paperwork and decides whether the case should be forwarded to the Professional Conduct Committee. This is only done when a conviction in the courts may call continuing registration into question (murder, fraud or indecency are examples) or where a charge may involve serious professional misconduct (such as failing to visit, treat or refer appropriately or taking sexual or financial advantage of a patient); a further and important consideration is whether there is adequate evidence to make the charge stick. The Conduct Committee (or more precisely a panel of about eleven people, including formerly one but now two laypeople, drawn from the members of that committee) hear the charges in public. The Council and the respondent doctor are legally represented.

Various disposal decisions are available to the Committee. At the most serious it may order erasure. Normally this takes effect after twenty-eight days; in very serious cases the Committee may order erasure forthwith. The Committee may suspend registration for a defined period; it may attach conditions to continued registration, such as limitations on the type of practice which may be undertaken; more recently retraining is sometimes suggested. It may admonish and conclude the case. Or it may find serious misconduct not proved and consequently conclude the case. After ten months, those erased may apply to the Conduct Committee for restoration to the register: of forty applications in the four years before 1987 and 1990, ten were granted, one adjourned and twenty-nine refused.

The Council receives many more complaints than ever come before the committees; most are dismissed or dealt with informally. The *GMC Annual Report for 1988*, for example, states that 967 cases were reported for the period 1 September 1987 to 31 August 1988. Of these, 760 included no evidence of a conviction, 'nor was any question of serious professional misconduct considered to arise'; sixty-six were redirected to appropriate NHS authorities on the grounds that they concerned treatment or lack of it under the NHS; eighty consultations were held with a view to informal action being taken, that is, a letter of advice (effectively a warning) being sent. One hundred and twenty-seven doctors were referred to the Preliminary Proceedings Committee out of the original 967 cases.

During 1987–8 127 doctors, involving 143 cases of conviction or serious professional misconduct, were brought before the Preliminary Proceedings Committee for their convictions to be considered (sixty-five, that is, over half) or for alleged serious professional misconduct (sixty-three); one doctor fell in both categories. Of the total, no action was taken in ten cases; sixty-four received advice, caution or admonition; twenty cases were adjourned; none was referred to the Health Committee (but some had been referred for health inquiries); thirty-three were referred to the Professional Conduct Committee.

In the same period forty doctors came before the Professional Conduct Committee, with a total of fifty-two cases of convictions or charges of serious professional misconduct among them; forty-three of these had been referred in 1988, nine earlier. Of the forty doctors, eleven were found not guilty of serious professional misconduct and their cases concluded. Six of the twenty-four found guilty were admonished and their cases concluded. Of the remaining guilty, six were erased, two forthwith; eleven were suspended; registration conditions were imposed on two; one was referred to the Health Committee; and one case was adjourned. In all, nineteen of the forty doctors had their cases concluded without any change to their registration status.

This example from the later 1980s is not untypical of the period I examined in my research in that no more than a small number of complaints ever reach the formal procedures. The pattern has continued into the 1990s. From 1 September 1991 to 31 August 1992, 1,300 complaints or information (e.g. about a conviction in the courts) were received, of which 123 (9.5 per cent) were dealt with by the Preliminary Proceedings Committee, who referred twenty-four (1.8 per cent) to the Health Procedures and thirty-four (2.6 per cent) to the Professional Conduct Committee. These last are the only ones which come into the public domain (Report of the Preliminary Proceedings Committee to Council, November 1992: mimeo).

In 1992, the Professional Conduct Committee dealt with forty-three cases: four doctors were erased; thirteen suspended (of which one was suspended immediately); six had conditions attached to their registration; nine were admonished or the case concluded; nine were found not guilty of serious professional misconduct; and two remained to be heard.

One gets the sense that the cases which get through are 'pour encourager les autres' rather than effectively to comb out incompetent doctors. Rosenthal (1987: 115) has explained the relative stability over time by suggesting the GMC limits the cases it deals with in light of its resources. Thinking of the extensions of disciplinary work now being proposed a retiring member, Dr Fry, has asked 'how much more will the medical profession be prepared to pay for an independent autonomous GMC?' (*GMC Annual Report for 1991*: 4).

There have, however, been two periods when the disciplinary activity of the Council markedly increased. One was in 1961 when Lord Cohen first became president and stirred a largely dormant Council to its disciplinary responsibilities. The average number of days a year the disciplinary committee met rose from an average of just under six in 1955–61 to sixteen in

1962–73 and to twenty-one from the time when Sir John (now Lord) Richardson took over until the Council was reformed in 1979. The number of days again increased noticeably in the 1980s. In the period from 1982 to 1988, the average had reached forty-three and a half days a year (collated in Stacey, 1992a: 140). In 1990, panels of the Professional Conduct Committee sat for seventy-seven days, a figure inflated by the thirty-six days spent dealing with the notorious kidney transplant allegations that live Turkish donors were paid for supplying kidneys to persons receiving private treatment in the United Kingdom whom the donors did not know. Of the three doctors involved, all were found guilty of serious professional misconduct, one was erased and two had restrictions placed upon their practice (*GMC Annual Report for 1990*: 19).

While at the most abstract level the interests of profession and of patients are one, in practice some disciplinary offences have a more immediate impact on professional colleagues while others affect patients more. For example, taking advantage of a patient for sexual purposes or financial gain, while reflecting badly on the profession if made public, are indubitably offences against the patient perpetrated in the treatment situation. Advertising and canvassing, on the other hand, are offences against the profession (the Monopolies and Mergers Commission insisted in 1989 that the tight regulations against advertising be slackened in the public interest) as are deprecating colleagues and improper delegation (see Stacey, 1992a: 155–7).

Furthermore, looking over a period of time at how cases were disposed of, offences against the profession were taken more seriously than offences against patients, although this has begun to change in the last decade. Not only is there more disciplinary activity nowadays than there used to be, more attention proportionately is paid to offences against patients.

I examined in detail cases at the various stages of the procedure for the periods from 1976–80 and 1983–9 (Stacey, 1992a: 150–68). During the 1980s more cases of a clinical nature, or bordering on the clinical, came before the Professional Conduct Committee than in the 1970s. However, looking at the larger categories of offence, it became clear that in the 1980s the Committee experienced the greatest difficulty in finding serious professional misconduct in cases of disregard of professional responsibility. More cases were found guilty when it came to dishonesty or non-*bona fide* prescribing (i.e. the misuse of controlled and dangerous drugs) (Stacey, 1988: 165–6).

A number of factors led to this difference. In many of the last two categories the courts will have found guilt and convicted, so the Committee has only to decide whether the offence calls registration into question, whereas in cases of possible serious professional misconduct the Committee itself has to find guilt. Members of Council have always considered it most important that respondent doctors should be treated with compassion – however sternly they might from time to time have to be reprimanded. All members, and especially those in daily professional practice, feel that 'there but for the grace of God go I'. The practitioner's perspective is inevitably different from that of the patient.

In my book I describe some imaginary cases, but invented on the basis of experience (Stacey, 1992a: 147–8). Imagine a doctor, a man who failed to visit and treat some children when called. The defence counsel attempted to put the blame on the mothers (whom he handled very roughly). The tough verdict that the respondent doctor was guilty of serious professional misconduct prevailed because of the insistence of senior doctors on the panel that it was the doctor's not the mother's business to diagnose. (The exclusive right to diagnose is jealously guarded and any wavering might create an awkward precedent.) However, surprisingly the Committee found admonishment a sufficient punishment; surprisingly because it seemed a most lenient verdict for actions which had put children's lives at risk. In the chairperson's view in a case like that admonishment is sufficient because the doctor had already been punished enough, having been fined by the local practitioner committee and having had the case hanging over his head for three years (so had the mothers).

In another imaginary example a great deal of convincing evidence suggested that a doctor had not only failed to visit and treat, but had written a prescription on the basis of telephoned information: the dose prescribed proved lethal. Furthermore, the doctor had tried to destroy the evidence and influence the coroner. Apparently a caring sort of GP, he could have been a friend. More so than most, from a practitioner's point of view this sort of case was one where 'there but for the grace of God'; a doctor's nightmare perhaps, but a patient's worst terror.

In cases like that proving the facts always presented a problem. The (to me astonishing) verdict of not guilty of serious professional misconduct might have taken two and a half hours to reach; the voting was narrow. In cases like those imaginary ones I, normally a dove in disciplinary matters, was a hawk voting for conviction.

Clinical autonomy

A major reason for the reticence is the doctrine of clinical autonomy. This has contributed to the failure of the GMC hitherto to consider any except the grossest cases of incompetence as 'serious professional misconduct'. A ruling on a dentist's appeal has now made it clear that bad clinical behaviour may be serious professional misconduct. In my view it always could have been; what was lacking was the will.

Clinical autonomy, held inviolable until recent strong challenges, states that all doctors have the right and responsibility to decide about appropriate diagnosis and treatment for their patients. The doctrine also states that where a judgement does have to be made, as, for example, in a court of law where damages for bad practice are being claimed, the only people who can judge the appropriateness of the clinical actions taken are other doctors. Furthermore, any judgemental body should include a doctor in the same specialty. Kennedy (1987: 59; his emphasis) says that 'the law only ever requires the doctor to act in a way *other reasonable and informed doctors* judge to be proper' and that medicine is the only occupation to which this applies (see also Giesen, 1993: 648–52). Expert evidence may, of course, differ (Havard, 1989).

Fitness and competence

The Council's task is to ensure that the doctors whose names it retains on the register are fit to practise. In Merrison's terms the 'maintenance of a register of the competent is fundamental to the regulation of the profession' (Merrison Report, 1975: para. 1). However, 'competence' is not the term the Council uses, but rather 'fitness to practise'. Nor is this merely a linguistic matter; Council has not hitherto addressed the area of competence in any direct disciplinary manner. That is to say, it has rarely defined incompetent practice as unfitness to practise.

However, unfitness to practise has been defined more widely since the early 1980s and especially since 1983 when Nigel Spearing introduced a Bill in the House of Commons which would effectively add 'inappropriate professional conduct' to the present charge of 'serious professional misconduct'. He proposed this after a case in which, although a doctor's conduct was so 'inappropriate' that it may have led to the death of a child, the doctor was not found guilty of serious professional misconduct. The notion of two 'standards' of charge did not find favour with the GMC. (Some suggest this was because the GMC dislikes any interference from Parliament. As Larkin (1992a: 6) points out, the medical–state alliance was specifically with the Ministry, now Department, of Health. Parliament could be a threat to both.) The New Zealand Council, similar to the GMC in many ways, does have a second category in addition to 'serious professional misconduct' along the lines of the 'unacceptable professional misconduct' finding suggested. The introduction of such a charge would mean that Council would have to take seriously and examine cases which at the minute are not forwarded because they are not judged to amount, or could not be proved to amount, to '*serious* professional misconduct'.

Reject the notion of two charges it might, but criticisms that the Council has not dealt adequately with incompetent doctors could, after the Spearing

Bill and certain other disasters, no longer be ignored. A working party was set up to examine the question. Proposals were made publicly available for comment in May 1992 before decision in November. Conceived soon after Spearing first put his Bill before the House, this idea, like all other proposals which emanate from the Council, has been the subject of much informal negotiation behind closed doors.

Still shying away from the term competence, Council is speaking instead of powers to review 'performance' in cases where complaints suggest a doctor's fitness to practise over a period of time is called into serious doubt. One of the points which the GMC continually makes in disciplinary matters is that it is only concerned with *serious* cases of misconduct or *serious* cases of impaired health. Only serious failures, it is argued, should affect a doctor's registration.

The performance procedure would operate rather like the Health Committee procedures. That is to say, where there is evidence that a doctor's general performance may be below par, as opposed to a single episode in which things have gone wrong, the doctor would be invited to submit to a review of her or his practice. These reviews would take place partly at the doctor's place of work and in any event hearings would be arranged in the locality. As a result respondent doctors would, if necessary, be advised of changes they need to make, and be recommended perhaps to go for retraining. They would not appear before a formal committee at the GMC headquarters unless they refused to submit to a review or to comply with the advice.

This proposal might have the positive effect of making discipline applicable to doctors whose practice may be detrimental to the public but who at present slip through the net. Unlike the Spearing proposals, the cases dealt with in this way would not face the same public scrutiny as do the cases of those at present charged with serious professional misconduct. The absence of clear criteria as to which complaints would go which way is also worrying (Stacey, 1992c).

IS THE GMC A GOOD MODEL?

The evidence presented here suggests those who are thinking of using the GMC as a model might bear the following in mind. First, the GMC has greatly benefited biomedicine, its practitioners' standard of life and security of employment. These benefits have largely derived from the state–medical alliance of which the GMC is the crucial medical ingredient. Second, the status of biomedicine and its practitioners has been achieved by (a) excluding healers of other modalities from privileges; (b) establishing a division of state-registered health labour which subordinates other health care professions to biomedicine. Third, the characteristics of professional self-regulation, even in the most high-minded and ethically thoughtful persons, tend to lead, probably inevitably, to biases in favour of the profession rather than the public; they also tend to conservative modes of regulation because of the need to keep the profession together.

The case of osteopathy

Osteopathy sought state recognition in 1936 when a Bill came before the House of Lords; at that time it was strongly opposed by the biomedical profession and defeated (King's Fund, 1991; Larkin, 1992a, 1992b). An essentially similar Bill put forward in 1992 was supported by biomedicine, nursing and physiotherapy – so this time an Act ensued. The Bill had followed a King's Fund Working Party report which, to impress its point that osteopathy should be accorded state registration, included the draft of a possible Bill (King's Fund, 1991: endpiece).

The Working Party was chaired by a Lord Justice of Appeal and included: four registered medical practitioners, one also a practising osteopath; two other osteopaths; and a health journalist. The Department of Health (DH) sent two observers, one medical, one non-medical. The secretary was a retired non-medical civil servant. The biomedical practitioners were highly placed men (*sic*): a past president of the GMC, a past president of the Royal College of Surgeons and an emeritus professor of neurology. It was Walton of Detchant who powerfully led the Bill through the Lords. Of the ten (seven members, two observers and the secretary) three were women: one osteopath, the health journalist and the DH senior medical officer. Seemingly none came from ethnic minorities.

The General Osteopathic Council (GOC), now to be established, will include twelve elected osteopaths, four representatives of osteopathic educational institutions with, appointed by the Privy Council, a further eight, seven non-osteopaths, so-called 'lay', and a registered medical practitioner (two initially). The GOC is closely modelled on the GMC with regard to functions and committee structure. It must keep a statutory register, establish qualifications for entry to the register, maintain conduct and discipline and examine complaints, directing them where necessary either to a health or a professional conduct committee.

There are some significant differences. 'Incompetent practice' is named as an explicit reason for disciplinary investigations (Malcolm Moss, Hansard HC, 15.1.93, vol. 216: 1179–80; Maxwell, 1993). The GOC registrar may order immediate suspension – a power unique among registrars of regulatory councils (Hansard HC, 7.5.93, vol. 224: 416). Government sees the GOC as a new model for regulatory bodies. Perhaps not insignificantly, the GMC is now considerably increasing its lay representation.

A major difference between osteopathy and biomedicine remains. The Working Party emphasized 'that our recommendations . . . do not provide for osteopaths to practise in the National Health Service' (King's Fund, 1991: iii–iv). Nor is this to be the case. The restriction to the private sector means osteopaths will not be subordinated within a biomedically dominated division of labour as were the midwives, nurses and other health professions. Have the biomedical leaders, in accepting the right of osteopaths to diagnose and treat their own cases, said 'thus far and no further'? Or do the osteopaths prefer the private practice restriction to biomedical domination? However that may be, the relationship of osteopathy to the state changed when the Bill received the royal assent on 1 July 1993.

The interests involved

Three sets of interests have emerged in the accounts given in this chapter so far: those of the healing occupations; of the patients and potential patients, that is, the 'public'; and of the state. Their interests, however, are not static over time: the problems faced by the state change, as do the goals of governments; new healing modalities develop, old ones are imported or revived; the felt needs and demands of patients and potential patients change. In order to assess the value and limitations of the GMC as a model for other healing modes I propose to look at each of these interests in turn.

1 The state

The power of the state through legislation and policy sets the framework within which healers may practise and clients' choice be enhanced or limited. The state is interested in having a healthy population, minimally for reasons of social order. It has responsibility for the protection of clients from exploitation. Furthermore, when the state is funding parts of the nation's health care it also has interests in the accountability of the practitioners in terms of costs as well as outcomes of treatment.

As the activities of the state expanded in the nineteenth century so did the opportunities for biomedicine – notably through developing state concern for public health including control of epidemics. The even greater expansion of state involvement during the twentieth century to include the direct provision of health and welfare services increased the advantages to biomedicine of their alliance with the state. However, the situation has now changed in two ways.

First, the accession of the United Kingdom to the EC puts pressure on government in terms of the free movement of health labour and the harmonization of training and qualifications. In a sense the 'state' has extended beyond the national boundaries. Variations in the way biomedicine is controlled and the very different – and less libertarian – status accorded to non-biomedical healing modes in Europe have to be taken into account in government policy. Second, government policies since 1979 have included a reduction in state activities (at the same time as there has, paradoxically, been a marked increase of central control). Along with this has gone the anti-monopolistic stance challenging the power of the professions as never before. Furthermore, apparently pro-consumer policies have been pursued, including consumer freedom, consumer rights and through them presumably consumer protection.

The scene has consequently changed for all modalities including biomedicine itself. The state ranks its alliance with biomedicine less high than formerly; recent governments have been less impressed with the GMC than were their predecessors. I mentioned earlier the insistence of the Monopolies and Mergers Commission that restrictions on advertising be reduced. While I have been told authoritatively that the GMC asked for more lay members on Council 'because we realized we needed them', my hunch is that the Council was at least strongly 'encouraged' in this project by ministers, whether through the agency of the Privy Council or the Chief Medical Officer. As Gerald Larkin points out:

> The state no longer is limited to one managing agency, . . . medical monopolies . . . may be seen to be part of contemporary problems rather than vehicles for their resolution. *The medical–ministry alliance has been displaced . . . by an extension of a new occupational class, the custodians of cost control and performance management.*
>
> (Larkin, 1992b: 10; my emphasis)

The public has been turning over the past ten to fifteen years to an increasing array of non-orthodox practitioners and this although much NHS treatment remains free at the point of delivery while most other modalities are only available privately. Such modalities have received royal patronage: the Prince of Wales played a part in the establishment of the King's Fund Osteopathy Working Party among other interventions he has made on behalf of the plurality of unrecognized healing modes. The notion of choice and a free market fits better with government support for a system of plural healing modalities than with the biomedical monopoly. In this case the question for the state is: how best to regulate a plurality of healing modes? And what method might be compatible with directives likely to emerge from Brussels?

2   *The healing occupations*

Among the many and varied healers at present without state registration, there is a good deal of confusion about the issues involved. Attitudes range from occupations, such as osteopathy, the majority of whose members are in favour of registration, to those which are opposed, such as homoeopathy; the many in-between are ambiguous (ACHCEW, 1989: 15–16; Sharma, 1992a: 183–7). Looked at from occupations' perspectives, what their stance should be crucially depends on what their goal is. What do they want to achieve?

Since each of the healing modes has its own understanding of what the healing process is and of the work it is doing, the lessons each can learn from the GMC will differ. The advantages to be gained, the compromises to be accepted, are likely to balance out differently (cf. West, 1992: 206–10). For example, historically the price for state recognition has been subordination to biomedicine. Is that an appropriate price to pay for a niche in the Establishment? What advantages might be gained?

A radical view on an allied issue is found in comment from Julius Roth (n.d.) on a proposal from the Californian Department of Consumer Affairs (AB 1896) to license midwives. Midwives had been rendered illegal in the United States in the course of the struggle with doctors, rather than being licensed in an inferior role as they were in the United Kingdom. Roth believed that with certification the practices of existing lay midwives 'would become more clearly illegal and subject to increased harassment' (n.d: 1–2). The medical control envisaged would be likely to stifle innovation and increase undesirable intervention in births.

Before considering the likely differences in response between the modalities, I should first comment on the advantages of 'a place in the Establishment'. There is no doubt that the exclusion of all except biomedicine from state-recognized educational institutions has worked to the disadvantage of other modalities (Fulder, 1992: 176–9; Sharma, 1992a: 96–7). Attempts have been made to redress this balance. The qualifications of the British School of Osteopathy gained validation from the Council for National Academic Awards (CNAA) in 1988. The Centre for Complementary Health Studies was established at Exeter University in 1986 and has now appointed to the post of Laing Professor of Complementary Medicine. The Centre offers degree programmes and undertakes research into a range of modalities.

How the various healing systems view the compromises which may be involved in Establishment recognition may well depend on the extent to which a modality feels that it is indeed complementary to biomedicine. By that I mean that while it believes it offers something unavailable in biomedicine, it is able to work with the scientific basis upon which bio-medicine theoretically rests. The osteopaths in the King's Fund Working Party are an example. Osteopathy 'is not an alternative to conventional medicine but a complementary discipline which offers patients an additional treatment option for certain conditions which can affect the body's framework' (King's Fund, 1991: para. 1; see also Sharma, 1992a: 180–2). Another modality may feel that its epistemology and cosmology are so different from those of biomedicine that it is truly alternative. Some acupuncturists seem to occupy such a position as do homoeopaths, so long profoundly at variance with allopathy. In practice I sense that many therapists and also the leaders of their professional organizations are not always clear about the implications of these differences in the bases of their knowledge and practice from those of biomedicine. Among other things such differences may mean that biomedical methods are not appropriate to test the efficacy of other modalities. Unravelling such problems may, hopefully, be a contribution which the Exeter Centre will make.

For those anxious that their therapies should be freely available to all, not just those with sufficient resources to buy private care, a different kind of tension emerges. Just how far are they prepared to go to gain a place in the NHS? Do they feel that they would be able to practise as their under-standing and training indicates if subordinated to a biomedical practi-tioner? Would their freedom and resources be compromised? Or will the new purchaser–provider arrangements be sufficiently extensive and also accord them enough space? The osteopaths will retain their freedom and independence to diagnose and treat as their training indicates at the price of exclusion from the NHS, thus also excluding the many patients who cannot afford the fee for service.

All modalities also face the question of protecting their practices given the threat of directives based on the less libertarian model of many Euro-pean countries where, with the exception of Germany, non-biomedical practitioners have less freedom than in the United Kingdom. Biomedical domination has made it difficult for British practitioners, for example homoeopaths, to gain recognition in Europe (Huggon and Trench, 1992: 245–7; on the German situation see Roth and Hanson, 1976; Unschuld, 1980). A state register may appear to offer protection in this context without any further advantages being sought, but it is questionable whether state registration as such is necessary or appropriate for this purpose. Huggon and Trench suggest that

> The easiest and, overall, the most satisfactory way is to ensure that all nonregistered practitioners belong to organizations which have strict codes of conduct and high standards of membership. This means they can protect

themselves and their members from accusations of malpractice and can demonstrate to the European Community (and, in particular, to the Commission) that there is no need for intrusive regulation from outside.

(1992: 248)

The British Acupuncture Accreditation Board, founded in 1990 with encouragement from the Council for Complementary and Alternative Medicine (CCAM), is currently seeking to establish a voluntary register of qualified acupuncturists. To this end the Accreditation Board has invited colleges which train acupuncturists to apply for accreditation: by February 1994 five major acupuncture colleges had applied and reached candidacy status; one further college has also applied. Younger colleges are understood to be waiting to gain greater experience with their students before applying. At present there is no suggestion of applying for state registration: establishment of the voluntary register is the goal.

What is clear is that if a variety of modalities are to gain state recognition in the United Kingdom or be required by the state to maintain registers such that potential patients may know who has had what training, then none can expect to receive the favoured place hitherto occupied by biomedicine, for that depended and still depends on a monopolistic position in which competition is restricted. State recognition may offer little more to the plurality of healing modalities than boundary definition. This, of itself, could turn out to be restrictive for those who use more than one modality in their practice, as, for example, an acupuncturist also prescribing herbal medicine (Fulder, 1992: 182).

The plurality of modalities may console themselves with the thought that the dominant position in the organization of health care formerly occupied by biomedicine is declining. Aware that the walls are closing in, biomedical leaders are following a tactic they have become skilled in, namely gracefully conceding ground when they know they have no choice, but manipulating the situation so that they concede as little as possible. After discussing the possible biomedical incorporation of acupuncture, Saks (1992b: 198) concludes that the medical profession has exhibited 'chameleon-like qualities' which have enabled it to be 'so successful to date in defending its interests against competitors in the arena of alternative medicine'. It is in the light of such understanding that I read the changing situation of osteopathy. However, as I have indicated, the osteopaths' solution may well be quite unacceptable to other modalities. In addition, individual registered practitioners are taking small amounts of training and offering these, for example acupuncture, as an adjunct to biomedical practice. This, as West (1992: 207) notes, is threatening to the modalities, which are being, so to say, pirated and 'medicalized' in this way.

3 Patients and potential patients – the public

From the public point of view the considerations are that patients and potential patients should have access to safe and efficacious services and that the practitioners should be trustworthy. If one healer or type of healer is not helping a patient, she or he wishes to be able to go to a different practitioner, perhaps in a different modality.

Historically the public were not restricted to one healing mode (Porter, 1989, and chap. 3 this volume). The people of Norwich in the early modern period had a wide array of healers of all kinds available to them including barber-surgeons, empirics and wise women (Pelling, 1978, 1982; Pelling and Webster, 1979). Well-informed and active, they 'chose freely among the range of practitioners according to their own and their friends' judgement of the nature and seriousness of their condition' (Pelling, 1985: 80);

> it is also possible to argue that the relations between doctor and patient were more evenly balanced than is the case today. Patients bargained with practitioners as in a commercial transaction and settled on an agreed product or 'cure'.

> (Pelling, 1985: 80)

A major argument for state registration rests on the assumed ignorance and gullibility of patients. Used as justification for the GMC, it is found again in the terms of reference of the King's Fund Working Party which refers to regulating 'the education, training and practice of osteopathy for the benefit and protection of patients' (and see King's Fund, 1991: para. 20). The asymmetry in knowledge has been assumed in the sociology of the professions. Johnson (1972: 41), for example, refers to the way in which the specialization in the production of occupational skill leads to the '*un*specialization' (his emphasis) of consumption. The patient's knowledge is experiential, general and unsystematic in comparison with that of highly trained professionals. This asymmetry provides a potential for control by the more knowledgeable.

The question is whether state registration does provide the protection for patients and potential patients which its proponents would like us to believe. Many assume it does (e.g. ACHCEW, 1989). Julius Roth is sceptical. He suggests that there is little evidence of the value of licensing practitioners in order to protect the public; indeed its value is negligible (Roth, 1975: 8–9; see also Roth and Hanson, 1976). The conditions of medical practice in the United States are of course different from those which have hitherto applied in the United Kingdom. However, my evidence about the GMC, outlined above, suggests that it has not been very thorough in protecting the public. The continued intransigent resistance of the British medical establishment to an inspectorate does not inspire confidence that it intends to offer thorough protection; nor do the professional biases in the proposed performance procedures.

Roth (1975: 8–9) further argues that the efforts to improve services and the desire to improve quality control within medicine at all levels are unrelated to licensing. This is also true for Britain: there are some long-established medical audit programmes inspired by the good medical ethic of providing a proper service (for example, in anaesthetics). Most, however, have recently been put in place as an urgent response to government blandishments.

At best one must conclude that, from the point of view of the public, the promised assurances that one may trust registered but not unregistered practitioners is over-stated. Professional self-regulation in the GMC, as elsewhere, is based on the 'trust-me' prin?iple. The claim is that experts know what they are doing and that their professionalism, derived from the collective undertakings of their profession, will ensure that they act to the best of their ability and in good faith.

TRUST AND ACCOUNTABILITY

I began this chapter by distinguishing between collective and individual therapeutic responsibility and have focused on the former. They are, of course, connected. There is no doubt that as patients and clients we have to trust our healers when we consult them. But how far does that trust derive from or depend on state registration? The question is whether state registration offers sufficient guarantee to patients before placing their minds or bodies in the hands of a practitioner. Furthermore, it may be argued that the 'trust-me' stance disempowers patients from taking charge of their own lives and health. The thrust of a number of modalities is, after all, to encourage clients to do just that. This is not to deny that practitioners are helped to honour this trust if, with their colleagues, they have worked through ethical dilemmas which may face them.

The formal regulation of professions takes place a long way from the treatment room or hospital ward; a long way from the interchanges between patient and practitioner (or between practitioners) which gave rise to the problem. In the case of medicine this is partly a matter of scale. The GMC had 188,936 doctors on its register on 15 October 1992 (Report of the Registration Committee to Council, GMC November 1992: mimeo). The necessary organization takes on a life of its own with its own problems and concerns (cf. D. Smith, 1987: 56–7; see Stacey, 1992a: 222–3). This is one reason why the best of intentions to protect the interest of the client become lost or distorted. The way complaints are handled all too often gives rise to further trouble, as any Ombudsman's report will witness. Even without its historical élitist legacy, the GMC would have difficulty in not appearing (and being) distant from the point of view of client and rank-and-file practitioner. These considerations do not, however, remove the inherent problems which beset professional self-regulation.

No legislation without investigation

One difficulty is that the principle of professional self-regulation, its advantages and disadvantages and how well it works, has never been submitted to public scrutiny. In the new situation, where the plurality of healing modalities active in Britain is now acknowledged, there is a case for examining and debating how much regulation is actually needed, how much protection and what sort of redress when things go wrong. Undoubtedly healers in all modalities must be accountable to their patients individually and to the law (see Sharma, 1992b: 21). The multiplicity of ways in which biomedical healers may currently be called to account is confusing (and time-wasting) for them; the many avenues of complaint and redress available to aggrieved patients, none of them altogether satisfactory, are confusing and daunting (see Stacey, 1992b).

My advice would be that the whole question of professional regulation should be thought through very carefully before any new pieces of legislation, whether relating to the GMC or to other health care occupations, are put on the statute book. This process would need to include attention to the best way to achieve space for *bona fide* practitioners of all modalities to work comfortably, for the public to have reasonable choice and also to be able to call miscreants to account, necessary if there is to be trust.

ACKNOWLEDGEMENTS

My gratitude to the ESRC, which funded the original research on the GMC (GOO 232247), and to the Leverhulme Foundation, whose Emeritus Fellowship has made this chapter possible. My thanks to Dr Phil Moss, research associate, whose research and analysis I have used extensively in this chapter and whose stimulating conversation I have enjoyed. I am furthermore grateful to him and also to Sarida Brown, Professor Gerry Larkin, Sir Norman Lindop and to the editors, Susan Budd and Ursula Sharma, for their valuable insights and critical comments on earlier drafts, and to Sarida for what she has taught me about complementary and alternative therapies. My thanks to Professor Gerry Larkin and Professor Julius Roth for permission to quote from their unpublished papers. Jennifer has continued to support and encourage me: many thanks to her for that.

REFERENCES

Note: References to the *GMC Annual Reports* and *Minutes* (pub. London: GMC) are cited in the text, except where reference is to an article by a named author.

ACHCEW (1989) *The State of Non-Conventional Medicine – the Consumer View*, London: Association of Community Health Councils for England and Wales.

Anwar, M. and Ali, A. (1987) *Overseas Doctors: Experience and Expectations. A Research Study*, London: Commission for Racial Equality.

Crisp, A. (1983) 'Medical Education', *GMC Annual Report for 1982*, London: GMC.

Fulder, S. (1992) 'Alternative Therapists in Britain', in M. Saks (ed.), *Alternative Medicine in Britain*, Oxford: Clarendon Press.

Giesen, D. (1993) 'Legal Accountability for the Provision of Medical Care: A Comparative View', *Journal of the Royal Society of Medicine*, 86: 648–52.

Havard, J.D.J. (1989) *Medical Negligence: The Mounting Dilemma*, The Stevens Lecture for the Laity, London: Royal Society of Medicine.

Horder, J., Ennis, J., Hirsch, S., Laurence, D., Marinker, M., Murray, D., Wakelin, A. and Yudkin, J.S. (1984) 'An Important Opportunity: An Open Letter to the GMC', *British Medical Journal*, 288: 1507–11.

Huggon, T. and Trench, A. (1992) 'Brussels Post-1992: Protector or Persecutor?', in M. Saks (ed.), *Alternative Medicine in Britain*, Oxford: Clarendon Press.

Johnson, T.J. (1972) *Professions and Power*, London and Basingstoke: Macmillan.

Kennedy, I. (1987) 'Review of the Year 2: Confidentiality, Competence and Malpractice', in P. Byrne (ed.), *Medicine in Contemporary Society: King's College Studies 1986–7*, London: King Edward's Hospital Fund for London.

Kilpatrick, R. (1985) 'Inspecting, by the Inspected', *GMC Annual Report for 1988*, London: GMC.

King's Fund (1991) *Report of a Working Party on Osteopathy*, London: King Edward's Hospital Fund for London.

Larkin, G.V. (1983) *Occupational Monopoly and Modern Medicine*, London and New York: Tavistock.

Larkin, G.V. (1992a) 'State or Professional Dominance: The Ascendancy of Orthodox Medicine in the United Kingdom', paper presented to the International Sociological Association conference 'Professions in Transition', Leicester, April.

Larkin, G.V. (1992b) 'Orthodox and Osteopathic Medicine in the Inter-war Years', in M. Saks (ed.), *Alternative Medicine in Britain*, Oxford: Clarendon Press.

Maxwell, R.J. (1993) 'The Osteopaths Bill: What it Means for Medicine', *British Medical Journal*, 306, 12 June: 1556.

Merrison Report (1975) *Report of the Committee of Inquiry into the Regulation of the Medical Profession*, Cmnd 6018, London: HMSO.

Moss, P.J. (1992) 'The Migration and Racialization of Doctors from the Indian Subcontinent', unpublished PhD thesis, University of Warwick.

Pelling, M. (1978) 'Medical Practice in Norwich 1550–1640', *Bulletin of the Society of the Social History of Medicine*, 23: 30–1.

Pelling, M. (1982) 'Occupational Diversity: Barber-Surgeons and the Trades of Norwich 1550–1640', *Bulletin of the History of Medicine*, 56: 484–511.

Pelling, M. (1985) 'Medicine and Sanitation', in J.F. Andrews (ed.), *William Shakespeare: His World, His Work, His Influence: Vol. 1. His World*, New York: Scribner's.

Pelling, M. and Webster, C. (1979) 'Medical Practitioners', in C. Webster (ed.), *Health, Medicine and Morality in the Sixteenth Century*, Cambridge: Cambridge University Press.

Peterson, M.J. (1978) *The Medical Profession in Mid-Victorian London*, Berkeley: University of California Press.

Porter, R. (1989) *Health for Sale: Quackery in England 1650–1850*, Manchester: Manchester University Press.

Roth, J.A. (1975) 'Recruitment, Training and Certification in Emerging Health Roles', paper presented to the American Association for the Advancement of Science, New York City, 31 January.

Roth, J.A. (n.d.) 'Comment on AB 1896', mimeo, Davis: University of California.

Roth, J.A. and Hanson, R. (1976) *Health Purifiers and Their Enemies*, London: Croom Helm.

Saks, M. (1992a) 'Introduction', in M. Saks (ed.), *Alternative Medicine in Britain*, Oxford: Clarendon Press.

Saks, M. (1992b) 'The Paradox of Incorporation: Acupuncture and the Medical Profession in Modern Britain', in M. Saks (ed.), *Alternative Medicine in Britain*, Oxford: Clarendon Press.

Sharma, U. (1992a) *Complementary Medicine Today: Practitioners and Patients*, London and New York: Tavistock/Routledge.

Sharma, U. (1992b) 'Professionalization in Complementary Medicine Today: An Overview', paper presented to the International Sociological Association conference 'Professions in Transition', Leicester, April.

Smith, D. (1987) *The Everyday World as Problematic*, Milton Keynes: Open University Press.

Smith, D.J. (1980) *Overseas Doctors in the National Health Service*, London: Policy Studies Institute.

Stacey, M. (1988) *The Sociology of Health and Healing. A Textbook*, London: Unwin Hyman (reprinted 1991, London: Routledge).

Stacey, M. (1992a) *Regulating British Medicine: The General Medical Council*, Chichester: Wiley.

Stacey, M. (1992b) 'Medical Accountability: A Background Paper', in A. Grubb (ed.), *Challenges in Medical Care*, Chichester: Wiley.

Stacey, M. (1992c) 'For Profession or Public? – the New GMC Performance Procedures', *British Medical Journal*, 305: 1085–7.

Unschuld, P. (1980) 'The Issue of the Structured Coexistence of Scientific and Alternative Medical Systems: A Comparison of East and West German Legislation', *Social Science and Medicine*, 14B(1): 15–24.

Vaughan, P. (1954) *Doctors' Commons: A Short History of the British Medical Association*, London: Heinemann (reprinted in M. Saks (ed.), *Alternative Medicine in Britain*, Oxford: Clarendon Press, 1992).

Waddington, I. (1984) *The Medical Profession in the Industrial Revolution*, Dublin: Gill and Macmillan Humanities Press.

West, R. (1992) 'Alternative Medicine: Prospects and Speculation', in M. Saks (ed.), *Alternative Medicine in Britain*, Oxford: Clarendon Press.

Witz, A. (1992) *Professions and Patriarchy*, London and New York: Routledge.

6   Therapeutic responsibility and the law

Robert Sumerling

My approach to the issue of therapeutic responsibility is that of a practising solicitor whose main experience in the past twenty years has been in handling the defence of several thousand professional malpractice claims against conventional medical, dental and midwifery practitioners in the courts and also in representing them in their defence against allegations of professional misconduct by their registering bodies. Not surprisingly, there is highly specific developed statutory machinery regulating the conduct of the conventional disciplines, and a substantial level of professional involvement both in the preparation and presentation of the defence of misconduct and related areas. I argue that this machinery can and should be used as a model in complementary medicine.

I am restricted by my own profession's rules of professional confidence in giving details of cases which could lead to complainants or practitioners being identified and so some facts have been altered in order to protect the anonymity both of complainants and of practitioners. So far, no distinct system of professional ethical regulation has appeared which covers all of the complementary disciplines, of which some fifty are described in the *Complementary Medicine Careers Handbook* (Foulkes, 1991). No form of regulatory council yet exists which covers all the recognized fields. As described later, some preliminary steps towards this aim have been taken by the Institute for Complementary Medicine.

The National Health Service and Community Care Act (NHSCCA) 1990 has resulted in major changes in the NHS, breaking up the uniformity previously imposed by the Department of Health. One of the main effects of NHSCCA has been to impose a purchaser/provider pattern on the whole service, so that in a few years all the conventional health professionals (except for the independent contractor general practitioners and dentists) are likely to be employed by health-providers in the shape of NHS hospital trusts and NHS community trusts. While the trusts so far formed are working to the same model, it seems likely that different trusts will evolve different rules (partly to suit local requirements, partly because of the personal preferences of the management) and become subject to a much looser central control.

Because the NHS is being split into a large number of semi-autonomous units (arguably in readiness for conversion to fully privatized health care PLCs), greater opportunities exist for complementary practitioners to enter the structure for conventional health care provision. Within the existing corporate structure, there exists a machinery by which complaints against conventional health professionals can be investigated and adjudicated at first level by management (to be followed in appropriate cases by warnings and dismissals) followed then by two levels of appeal, normally an appeal within the employer structure followed by an appeal to the Secretary of State. The most serious of such findings of misconduct in employment may then be referred by the employer for further adjudication on the question of professional misconduct by the conventional professionals' registering body, which is a topic I consider later (see also Margaret Stacey's contribution to this volume).

All the conventional health care professions have their regulatory bodies: the General Medical Council for doctors, the General Dental Council for dentists and the United Kingdom Central Council for Nursing, Midwifery and Health Visiting (UKCC). Between them, they impose statutory compulsory registration requirements on nearly all qualified conventional practitioners (there are separate arrangements for ancillary professions such as physio-, occupational and speech therapists and for radiographers). They set educational standards and also discipline their members. Such bodies provide a possible model for the organization of complementary practitioners.

In conventional medicine there are also a number of non-statutory craft associations such as the Royal College of Surgeons (others exist for physicians, radiologists, anaesthetists, obstetricians, ophthalmologists and general practitioners), all of which are recognized as playing a part in setting qualifying and practising standards. The presence of a universal regulatory body would not affect the freedom of individual professional skill groups to promote their skills and to organize their training. The theme of this chapter is that the controls existing in conventional medicine contain aspects which could validly be adopted in the complementary field to complete the bond between practitioner and patient. In contrast, anyone can practise so-called complementary medicine as long as they do not hold themselves out to be a doctor, or one of the other conventional titles which have statutory protection.

I examine the systems of professional conduct, employment procedures and malpractice claims in the conventional professions and discuss these in relation to the complementary medical sector. I also include a note on patient referrals from conventional to complementary practitioners.

THE CONCEPT OF SERIOUS PROFESSIONAL MISCONDUCT

All of the conventional professions define misconduct in different terms, though the intent is similar. Doctors and dentists can be disciplined only if they have been found guilty of 'serious professional misconduct', whereas nurses, midwives and health visitors are subject to a lower threshold of simple 'misconduct'. Nurses have traditionally been cast in a subservient role and can be disciplined for acts of far lesser gravity than those which would get a doctor into trouble. When I have defended nurses and mid-wives at the UKCC I have publicly commented on the irony that members of those professions can be 'struck off' for offences which might bring a doctor, at worst, a warning letter from the General Medical Council (GMC). The term 'serious professional misconduct' means: 'serious misconduct judged according to the rules written or unwritten governing the profession' (GMC, 1993).

The GMC has not produced a closed definition of 'serious professional misconduct' because circumstances change and its attention is continually being drawn to new forms of professional misconduct. It is said that:

> any abuse of the privileges and opportunities afforded to a doctor or any grave dereliction of professional duty or serious breach of medical ethics may give rise to a charge of serious professional misconduct.
>
> (GMC, 1993: 14)

I doubt that anyone would argue against that concept, but the definition has always struck me (and many others in the field) as inadequate because it does not deal with bad conduct which is less than 'serious', and so provides no way at present of checking it.

The way in which misconduct findings are put into effect by way of penalty or other orders has changed significantly in recent years. The conventional professions had only rudimentary controls until fairly recent times. They could erase a practitioner's name from the professional register in the case of misconduct, subject to a right to apply after twelve months for restoration. Since 1978, the GMC has been able to implement alternative orders by other means: admonition; suspension of the practitioner's name from the register for a period up to one year; and imposition of conditions on registration (for example, not to work single-handed or not to deal with certain areas of practice).

Since 1980 (under the Medical Act 1978) the GMC has had further powers to deal with sick practitioners without submitting them to a professional misconduct inquiry. Instead, the GMC has powers to impose conditions on or to suspend from practice where a practitioner's fitness to practise is 'seriously affected by reason of physical or mental impairment' (GMC Health Committee (Procedure) Rules, 1987).

In these cases, practitioners can be placed under voluntary supervision provided they accept they have a health problem, when they will then be required to submit to periodic examinations and to monitoring of their work. In cases where the practitioner does not accept that he or she has a serious health problem, a Health Committee may hold an inquiry and can then impose conditions on or suspend the doctor's registration.

The GMC at last intend to introduce 'performance procedures' for situations where:

> a doctor's pattern of professional performance appears to be seriously deficient – in other words so blatantly poor that patients are potentially at risk and action needs to be taken to resolve the deficiency and/or to restrain the doctor's freedom to practise.
>
> (GMC, 1992: 8)

Retraining procedures are envisaged with long-stop rules allowing suspension of registration where a doctor either refuses to cooperate in retraining or does not improve after retraining. Such a model might well be usefully applied in the complementary field.

The opportunity to achieve this reform has been available to the GMC ever since the last major reforms in 1978, when procedures to deal with sick doctors were enacted. The GMC has damaged its credibility both within the profession and outside it by waiting for so long. Even now it may be at least 1996 before performance procedures are introduced. The government currently has no intention of funding these procedures. The lesson for the complementary professions is that their standing in the public eye depends on the efficiency and impartiality with which they regulate themselves. The British Medical Association (BMA, 1993) argues for a series of regulating bodies for the various professions, a view with which I concur.

GMC cases involving breach of trust over treatment

There are sadly numerous cases in the GMC annals where doctors have promised cures for incurable conditions, charged large fees for treatment which itself is either worthless or of no comparable value, and, as a result, encouraged false hope but instead produced grievous disappointment among their patients.

In recent times, a number of doctors have been found guilty of serious professional misconduct for promising cures for AIDS. They have done so through private clinics which they themselves have owned, in which they have gone on to disobey GMC guidelines which require them to tell a patient of any financial interest they have in promoting treatment. They have in some cases gone on to give treatment for which they have been unable to demonstrate even an outside chance of success. The GMC has taken a very serious view of practitioners who thus prey on the vulnerability of the dying.

In a recent GMC case a doctor sold an expensive and ineffectual treatment to AIDS patients. It involved taking some of the patient's blood, separating the white cells, 'activating' the cells and transfusing the blood back to the patient. The doctor could not or would not explain to the GMC Professional Conduct Committee what the activation process was. He had been exposed in a television documentary after a journalist posed as an AIDS patient. The doctor was found guilty of serious professional misconduct and his name erased from the register – that is, struck off. It is obvious that such malpractice amounting almost to fraud should be heavily penalized.

Such a case raises the question of the machinery for disciplining complementary or alternative therapists who may also abuse patients, for example by having sex with them under the guise of treatment, and probably charging a fee into the bargain. In extreme cases such a therapist might be guilty of rape and/or indecent assault, but in many such cases the patient will be highly distressed and vulnerable and may be quite unable to submit him- or herself to the process of criminal law. In the early part of 1993 there was ample publicity in the media about such abuse of patients by therapists, in particular in the field of psychotherapy. The arrival of professional disciplinary and registration codes to which all therapists in the various specialities must subscribe will, in my view, be a move towards a mature system of complementary medicine.

Until such time as there are compulsory registration bodies for complementary practitioners, it may be possible for disappointed patients to try to invoke the criminal law against them by complaining that they had been deceived into paying substantial fees under false representation by the practitioner that a treatment could improve or cure their condition. In fields where 'improvement' and 'cure' are subjective and variable concepts, it could be very difficult to persuade a jury that a therapist's promise of benefit from therapy was fraudulently made if the therapist could show that the patient's expectations were too high.

If the practitioner has undertaken a careful consultation procedure (recorded in writing) which explains the possibilities and risks of the treatment, and if the patient then consents in full knowledge, it would be very difficult to sustain a charge of fraud.

Confidentiality

The GMC states that:

> Patients are entitled to expect that the information about themselves or others which a doctor learns during the course of a medical consultation, investigation or treatment, will remain confidential. Doctors therefore have a duty not to disclose to any third party information about an individual that they have learned in their professional capacity, directly from a patient or indirectly.
>
> (GMC, 1993: 26)

A doctor can only disclose clinical information about a patient with the patient's express consent. Otherwise disclosure can take place only if, for example, there is evidence of child abuse or if failure to disclose would expose the patient to risk of death or serious harm. In some cases, statutory rules require doctors to disclose confidential information, but unauthorized disclosure will expose a doctor to a finding of serious professional misconduct.

I imagine no reputable complementary practitioner would argue against this rule and that it should be possible to adopt it as a non-controversial part of professional ethical rules for the complementary professions.

Conclusion

My own experience is that the very fact of professional conduct proceedings can deeply distress and destabilize practitioners; I have represented many who have suffered deep anxiety, sometimes deservedly, when faced with them. Nevertheless, these proceedings can be very effective even if no order is made restricting freedom to practise.

NEGLIGENCE PROCEEDINGS

Where the bond of trust between carer and patient breaks down because the carer has failed to exercise proper care and skill and the patient has suffered injury, then the patient can claim damages for professional negligence in the courts. Malpractice litigation in conventional medicine has become a major legal activity, with an enormous expansion in the number of claims from about 1975 onward as a result of the increased public perception of consumer rights, and the climate of litigation in the United States, and with lesser public deference to the conventional health professions. At present, there seems to be little litigation between patients and complementary practitioners. A number of decisions appear in the law reports during the nineteenth century and up to the 1960s confirming broadly that an 'alternative' practitioner will be liable in negligence for injuries caused to patients in the course of the exercise of the practitioner's professed skill (Nelson Jones and Burton, 1990). I have not discovered any recently reported cases of civil negligence actions against complementary practitioners in the United Kingdom. This suggests that complementary practitioners have only a limited time in which to organize themselves to meet professional negligence claims.

If a patient is injured by treatment given by any practitioner, whether conventional or complementary, then claims can be made: (a) either under common law negligence rules for damages for personal injury; (b) under common law contract rules for damages for breach of contract; (c) or under common law rules for damages for assault. It may also be possible for the patient to make a complaint to the police authority of criminal assault and/or about deception.

Any relationship between a practitioner and a patient is legally underpinned by the practitioner's common law duty to take appropriate care and to exercise due skill to ensure the patient's safety as far as reasonably possible. This is merely an extension of the general rule of negligence that any person must avoid acts and omissions which with reasonable foresight are likely to cause injury to another. The existence of this universal duty to avoid acts or omissions likely to injure another person is often misunderstood or overlooked through the building up of case law in particular areas.

In conventional medicine, the law on malpractice has developed with detailed study of a range of issues, including: the standard of care to be exercised by a doctor when giving treatment (*Wilsher* v. *Essex* AHA [1988] 1 All ER 871 HL); adequacy of patient consent (*Sidaway* v. *Bethlem Royal Hospital Governors* [1985] 1 All ER 643 HL); the right of doctors to withdraw treatment from the brain dead (*Bland* v. *Airedale NHS Trust* [1993] 1 All ER 821); evaluation of damages for a lost chance of successful treatment (*Hotson* v. *East Berkshire AHA* [1987] 2 All ER 909 HL); the right of parents to control access to medical treatment (specifically contraception) by young people (*Gillick* v. *West Norfolk & Wisbech HA* [1983] 3 All ER 402 HL); the right of parents and others to submit the mentally handicapped patient to sterilization surgery (*F* v. *West Berkshire HA and Another* [Mental Health Act Commission Intervening] [1989] 2 All ER 545 HL).

Case law on negligence has tended to develop from the more dramatic cases; for example, the bedrock decision on medical negligence arose from an incident in which a psychiatric patient suffered physical injury when undergoing electro-convulsive therapy. The treatment had been given in accordance with the properly held views of a responsible and competent body of practitioners in the field in question and so was held not to be negligent even though opposing opinions were that the treatment as given was unacceptable. This rule, the Bolam test, might apply to determining liability in complementary medicine claims but is currently under challenge (see *Bolam* v. *Friern Hospital Management Committee* [1957] 2 All ER 118).

Complementary practitioners are unlikely to be involved in such crucial issues except that, for example, the issue of consent is central to any patient–carer relationship. One of the tenets established in the Sidaway case (cited above) is that there is a duty on a carer to warn a patient of any small risk that treatment may cause a very severe injury. Its main outcome is that a conventional practitioner should ensure that a patient is in possession of sufficient information about a procedure to be able to give a valid consent.

In the examples above, *Wilsher* was a claim on behalf of a child who suffered retrolental fibroplasia, an incurable condition of the retina causing blindness, and thought to be due to excessive oxygen given after his premature birth. The parents won their claim in the High Court and the Court of Appeal then dismissed an appeal by the hospital authority. The authority appealed to the House of Lords, which decided that the causative link between medical error and the injury had not been proved. The burden on the parents when the House of Lords then ordered a retrial can only be imagined, but in fact, at the time of writing (1994), the retrial has not taken place, nor does it seem likely to do so. The case can be seen as an indictment of the present fault-based negligence system. A no-fault system was first proposed by Pearson in 1976 and has been frequently discussed but shows little prospect of early introduction in the United Kingdom.

While detailed consideration has been given by the courts to the standard of care a doctor must attain, the duty of care so far required of a complementary practitioner is merely to act as stated above, to avoid acts or omissions which might be likely to cause harm to the patient. However, it can only be a matter of time before a plaintiff's lawyer argues that if complementary practitioners wish to be accepted as having the same standing as their conventional fellows, then they must achieve the same standards – for example, that it is not open to a trainee practitioner to escape liability because the problem was beyond them (part of the decision in *Wilsher*), but that they must instead undertake to hand the case over to someone more experienced or else stand to be judged as a practitioner who has claimed to have the experience and capability to handle a given problem.

I refer to the issue of insurance and quantum of damages elsewhere, but it is important to recognize that injuries to patients may include physical injury, psychological trauma and, in extreme cases, death. The practitioner's duty to avoid injuring a patient stems not only from the common law duty to avoid negligent acts, but also from the contract with the patient.

The courts will infer from a written or verbal treatment contract the implied condition that the treatment given will be competently performed, that it will be applicable to the patient's condition, and, subject to debate, but most likely, that it will be value for money.

OTHER LEGAL REQUIREMENTS

The somewhat misleadingly named Cancer Act 1939 (as later amended) outlaws the advertising of cures for cancer, diabetes, epilepsy, glaucoma and tuberculosis. The Consumer Protection Act 1988 (giving effect to the European Directive on Product Liability 85/374/EEC) places liability on practitioners who administer medicinal products. This liability comes into play if the 'safety of the product is not such as persons generally are entitled to expect'. The Supply of Goods and Services Act 1982 requires delivery of services – which will include complementary therapies – with 'reasonable skill and care'. The Control of Substances Hazardous to Health Regulations 1988 (COSHH) deal with infection from hazardous chemicals and body fluids. Therapists using invasive procedures such as acupuncture are affected by these rules.

PROFESSIONAL INDEMNITY

The Institute of Complementary Medicine (ICM) has, in my view, correctly recognized the fact that complementary practitioners are at risk of malpractice actions. Professionals who say that they make no mistakes delude themselves. The truth, I believe, is that most professionals make mistakes most of the time, but, happily, most can be rectified before any harm is caused. It is those mistakes which cause harm and where the mistake represents a falling below an acceptable standard of practice which entitle a patient to damages. I believe also that it is a minimum ethical requirement for a complementary practitioner to be insured against malpractice, which is indeed the position taken by the ICM. A practitioner who does not insure carries the personal risk of malpractice claims, so that his or her own assets are at risk. If the practitioner has assets, then he or she faces possible ruin by a single claim. If the practitioner has no assets, then there is every prospect that the patient will go without compensation. If the practitioner causes a direct injury of any severity or if there is a serious condition which ought to be recognized by the practitioner and referred for conventional treatment, then the figures involved may be substantial.

It is not my aim in this chapter to look at the values of personal injury damages claims, but in the personal injury field generally awards of £10,000 are frequent. Where an award of this order is made, legal costs in addition might be another £5,000 at a minimum. It is unlikely that many practitioners could meet that expense without, say, having to sell their home. On the other hand, failure to insure and inability to pay a claim (except perhaps by the practitioner paying instalments out of personal earnings over many years) must be seen as a negation of the practitioner's assumption of care for the patient. For any practitioner to 'go bare', that is, to practise without insurance cover, is, I would argue, irresponsible and fundamentally undermines the practitioner–patient bond. At a very minimum, the practitioner ought to declare to patients whether or not they are adequately insured before commencing treatment. The very fact that practitioners insure themselves increases the prospect of claims.

Many professional associations for complementary therapists, such as the Society of Homoeopaths, make insurance a condition for enrolment on their registers. The first way is on a 'claims made' basis, meaning that the insurance premium must be paid up on the date a patient makes a formal claim before the insurer will pay. Cover must therefore be maintained for at least six years after the practitioner retires or ceases practice. The second way is on a 'date of incident' basis, meaning that if the insurance premium was paid up at the date of the treatment challenged, then cover will be given whenever the claim comes in.

This is the merest sketch of professional indemnity requirements, but no discussion of the legal aspects of practitioner–patient relationships seems valid without it. In a society where medical and other treatments are seen as services bought in a market, they are bound to give rise to claims sooner or later.

None of the statute law or professional rules affecting conventional practitioners require them to hold professional indemnity cover. This is not the case in countries on the European mainland, where, for example, in Germany conventional practitioners are obliged to have professional indemnity cover as a condition of obtaining professional registration.

Professional indemnity is generally considered a poor risk on the insurance market and I would hope to see the complementary professions uniting to buy block cover for their own and the public's protection. I have not been able to discover any coherent information about professional negligence claims made against complementary therapists. The most expensive type of claim which might be made against a complementary practitioner is that he or she had failed to suspect in reasonably obvious circumstances that the patient was suffering from a disease which required the attention of a conventional practitioner. If a patient suffering from cancer delayed going to a conventional practitioner following advice from a complementary practitioner that the complementary therapy was sufficient, then the cancer might have progressed beyond the point where it could be treated. The patient would have a claim (and likely an expensive one) against the complementary practitioner for reduction in life expectancy and for the psychological trauma of finding that a treatable condition had become untreatable.

CRIMINAL LIABILITY

I have discussed the possibility of fraud charges being brought against practitioners who make exaggerated claims for their treatments and/or who overcharge patients. A significant number of conventional practitioners are charged each year with offences involving drugs (both controlled and non-controlled) and with sexual assault on patients.

Where doctors fall ill, it is not infrequent for them to resort to self-medication and, for example, over-prescribe controlled drugs such as morphine intended for terminally ill cancer patients in order to obtain an unlawful supply for themselves. I have encountered examples in the midwifery field where practitioners have secreted supplies of pethidine to self-administer and have then injected their patients with sterile water. Fortunately, such opportunities should not be open to complementary practitioners, given that they do not possess or prescribe conventional drugs.

I have seen a steady series of cases where doctors have fundamentally abused a patient's trust by indecently assaulting them. In some cases, general practitioners have pretended to carry out gynaecological examinations which have been no more than indecent fondlings for the doctor's own gratification, leading to distress and anger on the part of patients who, in many cases, believe the examination is legitimate because they cannot comprehend that a doctor would behave otherwise than ethically. In other cases, legitimate gynaecological examinations have been inappropriately prolonged and coupled with indecent suggestions.

In one case, a consultant psychiatrist admitted to having an affair over a period of months with a young patient in his care. The age gap between them was substantial. The affair was coupled with consumption by both doctor and patient of controlled drugs. The GMC took an extremely serious view of the case in striking the doctor's name from the register, stating that they did not expect him to apply to have his name restored to it.

In another example, a young doctor became deeply involved with a patient and an intimate, apparently consensual, fondling took place during therapeutic sessions. However, the patient was deeply upset by the way in which the interviews developed. The doctor was charged with serious professional misconduct but at the GMC Professional Conduct Committee was able to show that he had been left without effective supervision in fulfilling his role as a psychotherapist. The GMC found the doctor guilty of serious professional misconduct, but gave him only a warning and allowed him to remain in practice provided he confined himself to an area of medicine without any patient contact.

Other cases can be cited where doctors, both male and female, have formed genuine attachments to patients, very often in the course of the breakdown of either or both of the patient's and the doctor's marriages. The GMC takes the view that relationships formed within the context of a doctor–patient setting can amount to serious professional misconduct, although it is probably fair to say that it has endeavoured to escape its image of being more concerned with the doctor's sexual aberrations in this respect than with his or her failure to provide treatment.

In fact, many cases can also be referred to where doctors have persistently failed to visit patients or to give appropriate treatment and where serious findings made in NHS General Practice Service Committees have been referred to the GMC for consideration. It is likely that many more cases exist which are not referred to the GMC because the threshold for serious professional misconduct is high. It seems likely, however, that the GMC's *Proposals for New Performance Procedures* (1992) will enable more cases of unsatisfactory treatment to be examined than is now the case.

EXISTING EMPLOYMENT CONTROLS FOR CONVENTIONAL HOSPITAL AND COMMUNITY PRACTITIONERS

I propose briefly to set out the complex machinery by which the conduct of the great bulk of conventional practitioners is regulated. This machinery governs the National Health Service in the United Kingdom, through which the vast majority of conventional health care is delivered. The framework for the National Health Service is to be found in the National Health Service Act 1977 and in the National Health Service and Community Care Act 1990. Within this overall module, the conventional professions regulate themselves: doctors by the Medical Act 1983; dentists by the Dentists Act 1984, and nurses, midwives and health visitors by the Nurses, Midwives and Health Visitors Acts 1979 and 1992.

An examination of the rules for doctors who are employed by the NHS serves to show how the disciplinary model within which they operate might serve as a basis for setting up collective procedures in complementary medicine. I state this whilst knowing that at present most if not all complementary practitioners are working in private practice, often single-handed or perhaps at most in small partnerships, although increasing numbers work within the NHS. Conventional practitioners work either in employment in NHS hospitals, in employment in the NHS community sector, self-employed in providing general medical and dental services as general practitioners, or in purely private practice.

The first three groups come within the extensive regulatory rules both of the National Health Service and of their professional regulatory bodies. The fourth group, which may also include some members of the first three groups carrying out independent work, come under the regulation only of their own professional bodies.

The great majority of conventional practitioners work full-time or mainly under some form of NHS contract, either as employees (i.e. within the hospital and community sectors) or else as self-employed independent contractors (as is the case with general practitioner doctors and dentists).

Hospital and community employment and conduct arrangements

The conduct rules in conventional practitioners' contracts with the NHS deal with internal disciplinary mechanisms, and although they may be activated by an external complaint by a patient, they are more likely in my experience to come into effect as a result of internal action, for example because of peer complaints and management action taken as a result of concern expressed by other staff within a hospital or community setting.

The procedural framework by which the standards of individual professional conduct are managed within the NHS has remained largely unaltered in basic structure since 1948. In the employment context, procedures have to conform also with requirements of fairness embodied in employment legislation. Where alternative and complementary practitioners are self-employed, they will, of course, have no employer figure to whom they have to answer. The system I am describing would only apply when complementary practitioners are recognized by and integrated in the conventional health systems.

Hospital and community complaints

In 1985, the Hospital Complaints Act required all health authorities to publish and operate a system for dealing with complaints from the public. Various procedures for investigating complaints are laid down in Department of Health circulars. The Patients' Charter imposes service standards on health-providers, for example as to the maximum length of time to be spent on a waiting list, but it does not set professional standards. A patient who feels aggrieved at standards of medical care in a hospital is entitled to have his or her complaint promptly investigated and to be told of the result. In more serious cases, the provider may decide to hold a quasi-judicial inquiry either by having an inquiry conducted by a committee at which the patient can attend (with a lawyer or friend) and cross-examine the health professionals; or by carrying out an internal investigation followed by a written report.

In the most serious cases, for example in the Cleveland child sexual abuse case, the Secretary of State for Health can order a statutory inquiry under the National Health Service Act 1977, chaired by a High Court Judge sitting with professional assessors and with the full powers of a court to summon witnesses. It is hard to conceive how such a complicated and also on occasion extremely expensive mechanism for dealing with patient–carer breakdowns might be needed in complementary medicine. The ICM sees the need to achieve systems for dealing with patient dissatisfaction which are as effective as (though hopefully simpler than) existing procedures in public sector conventional medicine, and where the complexity of current procedures renders them less effective than they should be.

Complaints against conventional general practitioners

In conventional general medical and general dental practice, there are entirely different rules governing the statutory terms of service. These rules are in the National Health Service (General Medical Services) Regulations 1992. Similar rules apply to dentists, but although they represent the other major source of 'high street' health care, I will not consider them in detail here. The rules for doctors run to some sixteen A4 pages. Many of the requirements are straightforward and deal, for example, with the hours for which a doctor must be available for consultation. Central to the rules is paragraph 12, which sets out the kind and standard of service which a doctor must give:

SERVICES TO PATIENTS

12. (1) . . . a doctor shall render to his patients all necessary and appropriate personal medical services of the type usually provided by general medical practitioners.

(2) The services which a doctor is required by sub-paragraph (1) to render shall include the following:

(a) giving advice, where appropriate, to a patient in connection with the patient's general health, and in particular about the significance of diet, exercise, the use of tobacco, the consumption of alcohol and the misuse of drugs or solvents;

(b) offering to patients consultations and, where appropriate, physical examinations for the purpose of identifying, or reducing the risk of, disease or injury;

(c) offering to patients, where appropriate, vaccination or

immunization against measles, mumps, rubella, pertussis, polio-myelitis, diphtheria and tetanus;

(d) arranging for the referral of patients, as appropriate, for the provision of any other services under the Act; and

(e) giving advice, as appropriate, to enable patients to avail them-selves of services provided by a local social services authority.

I have quoted this rule in order to explain the complaints system which operates when the therapeutic relationship between doctor and patient has broken down and the patient wishes to complain about the general practitioner. I refer to this rule elsewhere in relation to the question of referral between conventional general practitioners and complementary practitioners.

General practitioners contract with the NHS through local units, that is, Family Health Service Authorities (FHSAs). The complaints system is regulated under National Health Service (Service Committees and Tribunal) Regulations 1992, which have existed in basic concept since 1948, though they are now under heavy challenge. Complaints can usually be commenced only by a complaint from a patient (occasionally from FHSAs themselves). Complaints are then adjudicated by a Service Com-mittee which has both professional and lay representation, followed by a right of appeal to the Secretary of State. The FHSA can 'withhold' pay from, that is, in effect, fine, a GP. A patient has a similar right of appeal if a complaint is dismissed, but the whole process can easily take two years from original event to final decision. Both the British Medical Association and the Department of Health are studying changes under which FHSAs would become largely autonomous in handling complaints and would be responsible for achieving their more rapid and often informal resolution. Doctors and dentists would be expected to attempt resolution of complaints under in-house procedures. One can see here a move away from bureau-cracy towards simpler and speedier methods of operating.

Complementary medicine equally has to move away from its present position where there is no system at all or at best only a voluntary com-plaints procedure. To gain respectability it will need to adopt uniform and compulsory standards for dealing with patient complaints.

Private sector conventional practitioners

In the private sector (comprising doctors who are either in full-time private practice or are conducting part-time private practice separately from their NHS work), the very nature of the direct carer–patient contract means that there is no employing body and no intermediate procedure for resolving complaints and grievances. This is likely to be the model for most complementary practitioners. Where there is a breakdown of the carer–patient relationship, then the patient has only two courses to follow: either to bring proceedings for professional negligence in the courts and/or to make a complaint to the GMC. Because all conventional carers must be registered with their professional bodies, a professional misconduct complaint can always be made whatever additional means of complaint may be available.

REFERRAL BY DOCTORS TO COMPLEMENTARY PRACTITIONERS

It has been argued that a general practitioner can refer a patient to a complementary practitioner in compliance with the statutory terms of service under the General Medical Services Regulations. I have quoted above paragraph 12 of the doctors' terms of service, where it will be seen that at paragraph 12(2)(d) the services which a doctor is required to give to patients 'shall include . . . referral of patients as appropriate for the provision of any other services under the Act'. Complementary medicine does not comprise 'any other service' under the National Health Service Acts.

The debate turns on the question whether a doctor must refer patients only within the area of conventional medicine or whether the duty of referral is carried out effectively if the doctor refers a patient to a complementary practitioner. Leaving aside the question whether referral to a complementary practitioner is effective in therapeutic terms, I believe it is correct to argue on behalf of a doctor that the terms of service are complied with if the doctor is satisfied that the referral to the complementary practitioner will allow the patient access to treatment which is likely to be as effective or more effective than conventional treatment.

Having stated this, I have never seen a case where a patient of an NHS general practitioner has complained because the doctor has either made a referral to a complementary practitioner without appropriate relief of the patient's condition, or else has refused referral to an alternative practitioner. There can be little doubt that at present refusal to refer to a complementary practitioner does not involve breach of the doctor's contract. It may be supposed that general practitioners who have an interest in holistic medicine are likely to be of an especially caring nature and hence their interest in complementary medicine means they are less likely to produce dissatisfaction among their patients. My researches elsewhere among the associations which represent general practitioners have revealed no case where referral to a complementary practitioner has been debated, let alone resulted in finding that the doctor is in breach of contract. (See also Peters's contribution to this volume.)

EUROPEAN DIMENSIONS

There are proposals to introduce rules which would require the provider of a service (this would include complementary therapies) to pay compensation to the consumer where the service is defective. A service would be 'defective' if it fails to match the consumer's reasonable expectations. A draft directive on defective services has been in circulation for several years but has not yet been brought into effect. If and when introduced it would be likely to have an impact on complementary practitioners (as well as, of course, on conventional practitioners), who would then have to prove the adequacy (that is, the appropriate level of safety) of their therapies in order to avoid paying compensation. As the proposals are drawn at present, this might well require the therapist to prove that there was no fault, while at the moment it is the patient who has to prove fault. For the great majority of practitioners who work carefully and competently the rules might make no difference, but they would be very likely to lead to more formalized patterns of treatment undertaken with the aim of protecting the practitioner. In turn we can expect an increase in the cost of insurance. The interface between these defective service rules and the existing product liability rules noted earlier in the chapter can only be defined when the new rules are made.

CONCLUSION

In this chapter I have outlined the way in which the mature, conventional medical systems are currently regulated. This can act as a baseline for the direction in which the unregulated areas of complementary medicine should develop. In order to protect the public and maintain their own reputation, practitioners in complementary medicine must evolve their own supervisory systems which at least match the efficiency of those of their counterparts in the conventional sphere.

REFERENCES

BMA (1993) *Complementary Medicine: New Approaches to Good Practice*, Oxford: Oxford University Press.
Foulkes, J. (1991) *Complementary Medicine Careers Handbook*, London: Headway.
GMC (1992) *Proposals for New Performance Procedures*, London: GMC.
GMC (1993) *Professional Conduct and Discipline: Fitness to Practise*, London: GMC.
GMC Preliminary Proceedings Committee and Professional Conduct Committee (Procedure) Rules, Order of Council (1987) SI 1988 No. 2255; GMC Health Committee (Procedure) Rules, Order of Council (1987) SI 1987 No. 2174.
Nelson Jones, A. and Burton, F. (1990) *Medical Negligence Case Law*, London: Fourmat.

Part III
Voices of the practitioners

7 Transference revisited

Susan Budd

In the autumn of 1900, a 17-year-old girl was brought by her father to see Sigmund Freud. Her real name was Ida Bauer, but she has passed into history as Dora, the pseudonym that Freud gave to her (Freud, 1905). Dora was the daughter of a wealthy, ailing textile-manufacturer whom Freud had treated for syphilis six years previously. Her elder brother, Otto Bauer, was to become a socialist theoretician and, briefly, Foreign Minister of Austria. Dora's father told Freud that his daughter had been suffering from recurrent neurotic symptoms since the age of 8 – depression, a recurrent limp, a nervous cough, loss of voice – and had been treated unsuccessfully by many doctors, to whom she had been sent against her will. He had insisted that his daughter accompany him to see Freud after he had found a suicide-note inside her desk, and, following an argument with him, she had had some kind of hysterical seizure.

Dora's father also told Freud that his daughter's latest symptoms had begun when Herr K., the husband of his mistress, had made sexual advances to Dora whilst she had been staying with the couple. The father, for obvious reasons, was anxious to stay on good terms with the K's, and Dora felt that she was being handed over to Herr K. as the price of his continuing to tolerate her father's affair with his wife. Herr K. had accused Dora of making his seduction attempt up, and she had been sent home in disgrace.

Freud took Dora into treatment. It was not a success. He strove to persuade Dora, partly through the analysis of two of her dreams, that her hysterical symptoms and amnesias were in part triggered by her un-conscious sexual attraction to both her father and Herr K., and consequent jealousy of Frau K., and that this overlaid in turn a homosexual attachment to Frau K., and to a governess who had been in love with her father. Her animosity to Herr K. was increased when another governess told Dora of his sexual advances to her, in just the terms that he had later used to Dora.

In keeping with his theories at this time, Freud believed that if Dora could acknowledge the real nature of her sexual feelings, her hysterical symptoms would vanish – as, indeed, some of them did. He pushed her hard to try to get her to accept what he said. His interpretations and reconstructions were brilliantly coherent and intellectually convincing. Subsequent commentators think that he bullied her, and her case-history has been held up as an example of both the sexual corruption of Austrian bourgeois life at the turn of the century, and the powerlessness of a young girl against an alliance of powerful adults, including Freud, all of them bent on getting her to stop rocking the boat.

As he wrote up the case-history, Freud was worried that his readers might think that he was putting sexual ideas into the head of an innocent young girl. Automatically, he turned to a medical analogy to justify what he was doing.

> It is possible for a man to talk to girls and women on sexual matters of every kind without doing them harm, and without bringing suspicion upon himself. . . . A gynaecologist, after all, does not hesitate to make them submit to uncovering every possible part of their body.
>
> (Freud, 1905: 48)

But Dora recast the relationship with her doctor in different terms. Like all patients, the main power that she had was the power to leave. After three months of treatment, she told Freud that she was going to do so. Freud felt that she was treating him not like a doctor but like a servant, the servant that she felt Herr K. had insulted. None the less, she left. She had turned the tables, Freud observed, and cheated him of the successful outcome that he felt he merited. Two years later she came to see him again with a new symptom – facial neuralgia. But this time, Freud refused her.

The psychotherapy students with whom I have read the story of Dora are struck by how angry Freud was with her. He wrote up her story with a hard-edged clarity and brilliance born of his frustration. But it is rare for anyone to be courageous enough to publish an account of a treatment which has gone so badly wrong, and whatever mistakes Freud may have made, he was still considerably ahead of his time in terms of doctor–patient relations. In England, an able young surgeon called Wilfred Trotter read *A Case of Hysteria* shortly after it appeared, and commented to his neurologist friend Ernest Jones that there was a man in Vienna who actually listened to his patients (Jones, 1990: 149–50). Jones was sufficiently impressed by the story of Dora to seek out Freud, and went on to train as a psychoanalyst and to establish psychoanalysis in Britain.

The enormous significance of this case for psychoanalysis was that it made Freud think about what had gone wrong. He had interpreted Dora's conflicting sexual impulses to her, but her condition had only partly improved. He put forward two reasons. The secondary gains from illness:

Dora's symptoms were her best strategy to retain any control over her situation. When, later on, emboldened by her analysis, she confronted the K's and made them admit the truth of what had happened, her symptoms temporarily disappeared. But in addition, her ever-changing ailments had been diverted by the analytic process: she had *transferred* her unconscious psychological conflicts with people in her past and present life into conflicts with her analyst. Transference, Freud had thought, was an inevitable nuisance in an analysis; he now saw that it was not just an obstacle to treatment. If it could be successfully analysed, it could be a means of cure.

In Dora's case, the clarity and purity with which the transference had emerged had been theoretically illuminating, but clinically disastrous. Freud thought that he had failed to analyse early enough Dora's identification of him with both her father and Herr K. Patients regularly form transferences to their physicians, and according to whether they feel that they are helpful and friendly, or antipathetic, they cooperate with their treatment or break it off. Freud went on to argue in his later papers on technique that all human bonds involve some element of transference. We never start a relationship *de novo*. We never love where we have not loved before. We bring to each new encounter our past experience, which conditions us to respond in various pre-determined ways. The metaphor that Freud used to describe the transference is the template. People slot into various unconscious patterns of expectation that we carry with us throughout life; very little is needed to trigger them off (Freud 1912: 100).

A commonplace example of this in everyday life comes with parents' visits to their children's schools. Most of us would ruefully admit that we find ourselves thrust back in our feelings to that time when we were children at school ourselves, and our real dealings with our children's teachers tend to get coloured by this. There's something almost Proustian about it; beneath all the brightly coloured drawings and projects, the friendly and informal teachers who look younger every year, lurks something older and darker. It's the smell, many parents conclude, that brings it all back.

As Freud pointed out, healers have always intuitively known about transference. They have used the fact that patients, in their anxiety and desire for help, transfer to them the obedient hope and blind dependence that they once felt for their parents and their teachers. In many healing encounters, this positive transference need never be disturbed. Michael Balint (1957), a psychoanalyst who was interested in helping general practitioners to become more aware of and able to handle transference phenomena, compared the meeting with the doctor to a drug. It was the most important drug the doctor had to prescribe, and yet the way it worked was little studied or understood. In this volume, Roy Porter describes how

quacks and irregulars also relied on evoking and using a positive transference, and Richenda Power and Gillian Vanhegan both discuss how they
begin to build up a relationship with patients which is based partly on
reality, but partly on unconscious transference elements.

Transference, Freud warned, carries a powerful erotic charge; the continued emotional contact, relief from intolerable anxieties, and talking over
intimate matters in privacy can lead us to fall in love with our doctors – but
also with our vicars, solicitors, professors, or other helpers and healers. The
seductive potential of this situation for both parties has long been known,
and creates the need for a professional ethic which limits the relationship
which healers may legitimately have with their patients.

To take an example. The New Zealand author Janet Frame, who spent
many years in mental hospital because 'a great gap opened in the ice-floe
between myself and the other people whom I watched, with their world,
drifting away', wrote a thinly disguised account of her experiences in her
novel *Faces in the Water* (1990: 10). Towards the end of the book, her
narrator, on the verge of discharge although by no means 'better', begins to
recover from the emotional thrall she has been living in and to notice how
the two psychiatrists, quite ordinary beings, are invested with extraordinary
power and significance by the patients.

> They talked to one another as if they were human, but their conversation
> fell strangely upon my ears, as if the mammoths in the museum had
> begun to speak.
> I still had the habit, more common in those who had been in hospital
> a long time, of investing the doctors' every remark and movement, and
> their families and their possessions with a wonderful significance, and I
> stood there confused by the very fact of their speech, and listening
> intently for prophecies and marvels.
> Dr Stewart was speaking. 'I can never keep a box of chocolates in the
> house. My wife has to hide them from me or I eat them all at once.'
> A commonplace remark, you will say. But I caught it and treasured it.
> (Frame, 1990: 234)

It is also true, of course, that psychiatrists and other doctors in a hospital setting
do have very real power over their patients' lives; in Janet Frame's case, to
move her between different wards, to give or withhold freedoms and privileges, to prescribe several hundred terrifying ECT treatments, and even to
consider a leucotomy. But psychoanalysts in private practice have no power of
this kind. Like Dora, their patients can and sometimes do choose to leave. The
power that is attributed to them comes from the transference.

One way of defining the purpose of a psychoanalysis is to say that it
aims to analyse patients' successive transferences to the analyst, to make

them aware of these, and thus realize how, unconsciously, they have always gone through life being afraid of, say, a certain kind of silent man, or feeling that they must look after someone who makes a particular kind of jittery appeal. It may seem bizarre that people who come for treatment complaining of things like impotence, insomnia, phobias or migraines end up being encouraged to talk about how they feel about their analysts, but in doing this we are not just egomaniacs. Partly, as in Dora's case, the physical symptoms fade away or seem unimportant; they are replaced by strong feelings of attachment and/or hostility to the analyst – the transference neurosis. Partly, psychoanalysts believe, the source of patients' difficulties usually lies in their unconscious expectations of human relationships, past or present. The psychoanalyst, by focusing them on him- or herself, draws their fire, so to speak, and so forces these bonds into the open. Why does this happen?

It is certainly not because the analyst is particularly remarkable or loveable (or malign or seductive). As Freud mordantly remarked, the physician 'must recognize that the patient's falling in love is induced by the analytic situation, and is not to be attributed to the charms of his own person' (Freud, 1915: 160–1). Rather, it is because of the abstinence on the analyst's part from continuously sending out all those messages that are part of normal human communication. In everyday life, when people talk to us about themselves, we react by advising them, reassuring them, telling them about our own experiences and feelings, respecting their sensibilities and the social conventions about what is and what is not to be spoken about, and above all emitting a stream of responses which tell them, by our words, movements, mood and expression, how we feel about them and what they are saying to us.

Analysts try to reduce considerably the number of messages that they send, and in doing so we breach many of the fundamental rules of human communication – by meeting questions with silence, by sitting out of sight, by refusing to divulge our own thoughts, and so on. Thus we arrive at a paradox. The bond between patient and analyst, which we hope will be the means of healing, is forged and intensified by the deliberate abstinence of one party to it. The abstinence creates a psychic space which is filled by the fantasies, conscious and unconscious, of each party about the other. The process can feel terrifying.

I hope that I have been able to carry my reader thus far without incredulity, because so far we can understand the transference in the terms that we use for ordinary human relationships. In the early stages of psychoanalysis, this is how the situation was seen; the analyst was to be as like as possible to a blank screen, to enable patients to project their assumptions on to us, and then to learn to differentiate between what we are really like and what they feel we are like. However, there is a stage in every discipline where it takes off from everyday common-sense, and becomes un-believable except to fellow-practitioners. But because all healing bonds contain strong transference elements, it may be possible for many healers to recognize what our more recent musings are about, even if they are not going to buy psychoanalytic theory as a whole.

The reader may well be feeling at this point that this is all well and good, but not particularly important. Psychoanalysis in Britain is a tiny pro-fession, with fewer than three hundred active members. Apart from a brief period around 1920 and during the last couple of decades there has been little interest in it, and what there is is often hostile and dismissive. None the less, psychoanalytic thinking about the nature of the therapeutic relationship has had considerable influence (Halmos, 1965; Rieff, 1966). Its most direct influence has been on psychotherapy and counselling – much larger professions, with six to eight thousand members each in Britain – and beyond that, on social work via the social casework movement, on child guidance, teaching, and on psychiatry. Much of this influence came not directly from Europe but from the United States, where for a time psychoanalysis was much more enthusiastically incorporated into the caring professions.

As with any body of knowledge which is adapted for social use, in the process much was abandoned, over-simplified and distorted. But it is still true that much of the thinking about the nature of the bond between patient and healer, and its crucial importance for treatment, comes from within the psychoanalytic tradition. If there *is* anything remarkable about good analysts, it consists precisely in their skill and sophistication in discerning what is going on under the surface of human encounters, in being at once part of them and yet detached, and able to make these deeper currents visible. The knowledge is rather uncomfortable; once we have it, we can never really live in the Garden of Eden again. Living with the knowledge is one reason for the notoriously prickly nature of politics in psychoanalytic bodies. Another consequence, which I will return to, is that it casts into question much of taken-for-granted reality, including our unquestioning assumptions about the nature of the relationship between patient and healer. In the remainder of this chapter, I first sketch out some of the developments and refinements within the psychoanalytic tradition in the concept of transference and its consequences for the therapeutic relationship, and then I revisit, so to speak, the concept of transference from a sociological viewpoint, and discuss the difficulties which psychoanalysis has had as a profession in both recognizing the nature of the analytic encounter, and yet allowing it to be a professional relationship just like any other.

Both these issues have revolved around the explicit and implicit comparison of the psychoanalyst with the doctor.

TRANSFERENCE DEVELOPED

One question that analysts are often asked is: do you think that there is any 'real', that is, non-transferential, relationship between the patient and the analyst? The classical view is that there is; that at the beginning and end of the relationship the patient can assess the analyst as realistically as anyone, but that as the transference takes hold, the power to do so wanes. At first, Freud and his followers hoped that they could work with patients to spot all the conscious and unconscious assumptions that were being made about them, and show that these came from within and had been projected on to the analyst as on to a blank screen. If patients could see this process at work in relation to the analyst, they could do so in their relationships with other people as well, both in the past and in their present lives, and at the end of treatment they should be able to deal with people freely, flexibly and realistically, and the transference would largely have withered away.

We now believe that a strong transference exists before patient and analyst meet for the first time; often we will be told in the first consultation that we are not what was expected, which comes as a great relief or disappointment. I once interviewed a young woman who had been sent along by her GP to a psychotherapy clinic. She had discussed it with her friend, who thought that the palmist at Camden Lock would be more use, but she thought she would try me first as I was free. After half an hour, she asked me if she was being hypnotized, or when would I start? Woody Allen has helped to form the notions of the more sophisticated. Several patients have told me how unwittingly influenced they were when they first came to analysis by the shrinks in the Hollywood movies of the 1950s. All this is conscious; it is the deeper fears and desires we bring that cause us trouble.

Part of the relationship between therapist and patient must remain realistic and cooperative – patients have to get themselves there at the right time, after all, and so must believe on some level that they need help and that the analyst is trying to provide it. This is sometimes called the therapeutic alliance or the real relationship, to distinguish it from the transference relationship which runs alongside, at times so powerfully that it threatens to engulf the analysis. It is also true that the transference can be more or less 'realistic'. The patients who see me as a housewife or a headmistress are making transferences which are more approximate to my own view of myself than the one who suspected I had been a nun because of my spiritual aura, or the one who couldn't look at the faces of the prostitutes behind King's Cross Station for fear he'd see me among them.

But as our views have developed, it has become harder to separate cleanly the 'irrational' transference from the 'real' relationship. Partly this is because of the nature of what we now believe is transferred. Freud talked at first as if what was aroused in the patient was adult eroticism. But his views on human instincts changed, and we came to see the experiences of very young babies with their mothers as more and more important. (Dora's mother scarcely figures in her case-history.) We now see more aggression in our patients, and more mixtures of love and aggression expressed in unconscious fantasies of relating to parts of other people; wanting to bite them, get inside them, expel them, stuff things into them, blow them into bits, and therefore the fear that other people, primarily the analyst, will want to retaliate in kind. We had these fears long before we could talk, and it's a struggle to get them into consciousness and speech.

The other change has been the growth of knowledge of and interest in the counter-transference, that is, the response of the analyst, conscious and unconscious, to the patient. This blurs any neat distinction between the analyst as representing the 'real world', and the patient's unconscious fantasy, and it also alters our conception of the relationship with the patient. Initially, true to the medical model, psychoanalysts thought that insofar as they were affected by their patients – moved to anger, disgust, love, hatred, fear, sorrow, laughter, etc. – they had failed. No longer could they be the well-polished mirror, the skilful surgeon, that Freud had advocated. Then several papers appeared around 1950 (Heimann, 1950; Racker, 1953; Winnicott, 1949) which argued that the analyst's counter-transference was not only inevitable, but also useful. The patient is trying to communicate something which cannot yet be put into words – the inner weather which has dominated much of their lives. The counter-transference, like the transference, is not a nuisance but essential evidence. The analyst's task is to try to disengage from responding within it by becoming conscious of it, and basing interpretations upon it. How this can best be done and the various ways it can be understood are the subjects of many current psycho-analytic papers.

This newer approach reduces the distance between analyst and patient. Now both parties have fantasies, conscious and unconscious, about each other, and affect one another. The patient can unconsciously scent a great deal about the analyst's state of mind, and the analyst must be very alert as to how he or she is actually feeling, and the ways in which the patient seems to be picking this up and reacting to it. We must also be aware of how powerfully we can be affected by our patients' unconscious projections.

The reader may well wonder what all this has to do with the idea of cure – a word many analysts are now reluctant to use. Some analysts believe that it is the real relationship between someone who is trying to communicate his or her state of mind, and someone else who is trying to understand it, that is the therapeutic part of the analysis – that interpretation is less important than being felt to be sincerely trying to understand and tolerate the patient's inner world. 'It is the physician's love which heals the patient', said Karl Abraham, an early follower of Freud. It is difficult to demonstrate that different schools of therapy have markedly differing results; whilst we may prefer our own theories, and consider others, past or present, to be wrong or incomplete, we all seem to have our successes and failures.

This is rather embarrassing if we believe that it is correct interpretation alone which cures. People who seem to get better because of their attachment to the therapist are said to have had a 'transference cure', which is sometimes dismissed as short-lived. I know of no good evidence for this. The situation seems analogous to the 'placebo effect' in physical medicine. There are few outcome studies of psychoanalysis, and enormous obstacles to designing them. The necessary confidentiality, the difficulty of defining improvement and in whose terms, the way people alter after an analysis and change their minds about it, the pressure that a follow-up would exert on both parties, are all reasons to be wary. The disappearance of physical symptoms might seem like a good criterion, but it seems that the offer of many sorts of help and treatment affects the auto-immune system. As therapists, we are likely simply to feel grateful that it does work so often.

Given that much of the time the positive transference works wonders, why don't we let it alone? Here different schools diverge. Counsellors do let it alone if it remains reasonably realistic; that is, if their clients go on regarding them as if they were friends, good parents or teachers, and don't progress to assuming that they actually are those people who will therefore see them on demand, tell them what to do, and so on. As we move across the spectrum from counselling to psychotherapy to Jungian analysis to psychoanalysis, we are more likely to find the positive transference being challenged. Here there is an important issue in technique.

Classical psychoanalysis is sometimes criticized for being too cold and austere. The patient, searching for sympathy, is met by someone who is reserved and objective. Many psychotherapists, and some analysts, believe that to behave in this way simply repeats for some patients the experiences they had in infancy with missing or unresponsive parents. The patient will go along with this, or, rather, a false part of themselves that has learned to manage will, but meanwhile the hope of finding a way to make a new start will gradually die. These views are often associated with Sandor Ferenczi, a likeable, gifted, tragic Hungarian analyst who was never really able to dissent from Freud until the end of his life. Ferenczi had been the analyst of Ernest Jones, Melanie Klein and Michael Balint, all of whom became leading British analysts. As in all analytic controversy, the disagreements over ideas and technique in Britain since the 1930s have been fuelled and amplified by the loyalties, jealousies and antagonisms that everyone feels toward their own and each other's analyst.

This issue, in varying forms, comes up again and again in psychoanalytic debate. It's connected with the question of real experience versus unconscious fantasy. Was the child really brutalized, sexually abused, and so on, by the parents, or was there an element of unconscious fantasy? Freud is often accused of saying it was fantasy; in fact, his theories went through three stages, where the first and last gave more importance to external reality. He also posed the harder question: what difference does it make? We are concerned with the patient's inner world, with how they see it. If acknowledging the reality of trauma and being sympathetic could cure, their friends would have healed them long ago.

Some extremely ill, out-of-touch people form a very negative transference, with little or no therapeutic alliance. They feel that the analyst is wholly bad, cruel, useless, overwhelming, seductive and so on. At some point, they become untreatable, but where that point is is uncertain. Freud felt that very schizoid, autistic people were untreatable because they didn't form a transference; we now think that they do, but of a very peculiar kind. The analyst is no longer experienced as a whole or consistent person, but rather as a jumbled series of fragments which the patient can't consistently locate inside or outside his or her own skin.

To return to the question as to whether the healing bond, in order to be therapeutic, needs to be a warm one. Many patients could not stand it. Their fear of human intimacy is so great, they feel so overwhelmed and engulfed by other people, so dangerous and endangered, that the slightest sign that the analyst has any kind of personal reaction to them is intensely frightening. The strict boundaries of time and etiquette of the analytic session are relieving to them. They will describe how jeopardized they felt when previous therapists smiled at them, told them anecdotes about their children, or prolonged the session for five minutes. We hope to enable them to relax the tight set of rules they use to protect themselves against all spontaneous contact, but until this has happened, warmth would feel far too frightening.

It was considering this sort of reaction that made Freud wary. It's no good, he thought, wanting our patients to see us as we really are, wanting to cure them, allowing them to draw us into a relationship in which we are the powerful benevolent person who is going to heal them. As Dora was, many patients are driven from doctor to doctor, healer to healer, pushing them to propose treatments which don't work, whilst they helplessly re-enact the frustrating encounters of their earliest years. 'What we do not understand, we are compelled to repeat.' Freud called this the death instinct. Whether we find this concept useful or not, the behaviour is perfectly real and is a problem for any therapist or healer – not to mention probation officers, social workers, those who try to treat addicts, and so on. Many of the anecdotes in Michael Balint's *The Doctor, His Patient and the Illness* (1957), based on his seminars with GPs to discuss their difficult or 'fat envelope' patients, show how they could not establish a healing bond with the doctor.

Balint talks of the doctor's apostolic function, the need to convert the patient to the doctor's beliefs as to how this illness, pain, etc. should be understood and borne. But at times of our own or our children's serious illness, mature responsibility is really a lot to expect in any of us. A serious criticism which can be addressed to both analysts and alternative practitioners is whether they do not at times expect too much of their patients. Both tend to imply that some at least of the patient's woes are of their own making. Both tend to stress the virtue, indeed the necessity, of taking charge of one's own life and illness.

It may be that at times this is just too much, and that the biomedical model in which illness has nothing to do with the mind is a kinder one. I have been impressed with the way that many people use knowledge of the psychic roots of physical illness to punish themselves and blame other people. Cancer, in particular, seems susceptible to being made into a moral vehicle. Because an illness is psychosomatic in origin doesn't mean that it doesn't hurt, isn't serious, or can be reversed by an effort of will; people die of psychosomatic illnesses every day. They are not the same thing as malingering. It is ironic that it is psychoanalysis which is used in this punishing way, for it began with Freud insisting that hysterical symptoms should be taken as having a serious meaning, since they were the patient's compromised attempt to show what was the matter and try to get well.

By this stage, it can be seen that the conception of the bond between therapist and patient within psychoanalysis has moved far from the original medical model. The analyst can't be a detached expert; the skill we use is much more intuitive and introspective. The relationship that we form with each patient is unique to us both – someone else would have done it differently, even if they ended up at the same place. The relationship is a more equal one, and is not supported by the rest of society and the medical establishment. In fact many patients seek treatment in the face of considerable resistance. The requirements for confidentiality are far more rigorous than they are in physical medicine – you'd mind public knowledge of the state of your liver less than of the state of your marriage – and so shared knowledge and joint diagnosis are not possible in the way that they are in medicine. Psychoanalysis is in many ways an extremely lonely profession.

Which brings us to our final question: What effect does this have on the social identity of psychoanalysts?

TRANSFERENCE REVISITED

If we look at the relationship between therapist and patient with a socio-logical eye, it is a highly peculiar one. What *feels* real is the transference relationship; what *is* real is that this is also a contractual relationship with a trained professional. The professional relationship is forgotten by the patient most of the time; the psychoanalyst has to be aware of it.

It is infinitely easier if patient and analyst meet as strangers; if neither of them have any contact with each other's 'real' life. Dora's case was a terribly compromised one. Her father had been Freud's patient; he brought his daughter along, demanding a cure for her in his terms. She felt he'd been evading the issue of his sexual behaviour for years, and dragging her along to various doctors instead. Freud was drawn in to advocating her father's solution to Dora. Now analysts search for anonymity, and find it convenient not to know too much about each other. But the profession has at times to have a public identity.

Initially Freud spontaneously likened the analyst to a doctor, and used 'physician' interchangeably with 'analyst'. But as he began to attract supporters the medical profession became largely hostile. Many of Freud's followers were laymen and -women who were keen to practise analysis. Under Austrian law, which recognized the right only of those with medical degrees to treat patients, they operated illegally. In 1926, Theodor Reik, one such lay practitioner, was taken to court by one of his patients.

In the same year, Freud wrote *The Question of Lay Analysis*, addressed originally to a senior government official who was interested in the issue. Despite his forty-one years as a doctor, he now thought that being a doctor had little to do with being a psychoanalyst.

> in this instance, the patients are not like other patients, the laymen are not really laymen, and the doctors have not exactly the qualities which one has a right to expect of doctors and on which their claims should be based.
>
> (Freud, 1926: 184)

He was bitterly funny about the ineffectual efforts of doctors to treat neurosis. Cures were hard to achieve in any case (this was before psycho-tropic drugs), but

> if a nerve specialist fails to restore his patients no one is surprised. People have not been spoilt by success in the therapy of the neuroses; the nerve specialist has at least 'taken a lot of trouble with them.' Indeed, there is not much that can be done; nature must help, or time. With women, there is first menstruation, then marriage, and later on the menopause. Finally, death is a real help.
>
> (Freud, 1926: 232)

Nevertheless, he could see the social power of the role of the physician, and that his new and controversial science was in need of its protection. Many of his analytic colleagues who were doctors wanted to exclude lay analysts; he noted their anxieties about being excluded and isolated by their medical colleagues, and their fear of competition. He conceded that doctors were needed for an initial diagnosis of analysands to exclude organic illness, but that after that psychoanalysis was part of psychology, and so needed different talents and training. It would be as irresponsible for doctors who hadn't been trained as psychoanalysts to treat patients analytically as for laymen to try to treat organic illness. (A point which is made about alternative practitioners in some of the other chapters in this book.)

His pamphlet led to a debate within the analytic movement about both the training and the admission of lay members. Most psychoanalytic societies have accepted lay members, some willingly. Some, such as the British Psychoanalytical Society, used to encourage them to train as doctors whenever possible, restricted the proportion of lay members until forced to give up, and still actively seek medical applicants. But the largest and most powerful society, the American Psychoanalytic Association (APA), only admitted doctors, apart from a few highly respected European refugees. Their reasons were complex: partly they were self-defence against various state medical organizations which legislated during the 1920s to exclude quacks; it was feared that if some lay analysts were admitted, the whole profession would be condemned as quacks. Partly they resented the dominance of European psychoanalysis – 'the Pope from Vienna' – and the economic competition from the growing numbers of non-medical refugees (Kurzweil, 1989: 50–3; 226–7). The profession remained medical in the United States until 1985, when a number of non-medical therapists successfully sued the APA and two of its affiliated institutes for practising discrimination and restraint of trade.

The nature of analytic training, centred as it is on the candidate's personality and on the development of intuitions and skills which are emotional as well as intellectual, means that it is difficult to integrate within any system of higher education. The criteria for the selection and success of candidates cannot be standardized or publicly discussed. The training is based on the training analysis and then seeing patients under supervision, and resembles an apprenticeship, with its emphasis on absorbing the skill of a master-craftsman by long and close association, rather than a university degree.

Psychoanalysis has had an uneasy relationship with British universities. It has appeared sporadically in various contexts, most recently in courses dealing with feminism, film and literary studies; a few appointments in psychoanalysis and its history have recently been made. Prior to that, it occasionally appeared in courses in psychology, sociology and literature; in a few psychiatry departments, interest was encouraged; above all, it appeared in a rather denuded form as useful knowledge for those training to deal with children, delinquents and the poor. There was a brief period in the early 1920s, centred on Cambridge, when it was seen as something educated people should know about. The Bloomsbury Group were interested in it, and at least four of them – James and Alix Strachey, and Adrian and Karin Stephens – became analysts themselves. But it has otherwise had a rather shadowy existence. Psychoanalysts find this quite congenial.

Conditioned as we are to anonymity, to being everything in and yet nothing outside the analytic session, being social non-persons feels quite appropriate. The cost of this to the profession is that we exist, with very rare exceptions, outside the system of state medicine and only in London. Many psychoanalysts work as psychiatrists, psychotherapists or clinical psychologists, but they are rarely able to practise psychoanalysis within the NHS. Although many psychotherapists acknowledge the importance of analytic thinking in their work, analysts on the whole avoid being thrust into the role of leaders or spokespersons for the profession, and this tendency seems to have increased if anything since the Second World War.

The dilemma for analysts, as for other alternative practitioners, is that if we work within orthodox medicine we may be forced to work in ways and contexts which are inappropriate for our own view of our knowledge and skill, but if we work privately, the length of treatment means that many people who could be much helped cannot afford it, or never find their way to us. The referral network is uneven. Some GPs are very ready to make referrals, appropriate or not; others do everything they can, according to the patients who finally reach us, to discourage them. In countries such as Australia, where some psychotherapy is paid for by state or private insurance schemes, this introduces a set of controls which can disrupt the therapy, and often such schemes will only reimburse therapists who are also doctors.

How did this situation – of a professional identity which is internally reasonably secure, but externally only partly recognized – come about? The psychoanalytic profession everywhere is affected by the public's anxieties and fears about a form of knowledge which is socially subversive and psychologically uncomfortable. In Britain, the profession was founded and run by Ernest Jones, and to a lesser extent Edward Glover, until the Second World War. Both doctors, they had to manoeuvre between falsifying psychoanalysis internally by defining it as an orthodox medical encounter, and yet using their medical status and political skill to secure a safe niche for it as a form of therapy which would be accepted by the medical establishment. In their tactics, we can see the complex interweaving and manipulation of attitudes to orthodox medicine.

Jones established the British Psychoanalytical Society in 1919, a journal in the following year, and a clinic for 'needy patients' in 1926. Psychoanalysis had attracted a certain amount of support by this time because simple forms of 'the talking cure' had proved much more effective than neurology in treating thousands of shell-shock cases during and after the Great War. But there were some anxieties. *The Times* occasionally reported suicides among those said to be in analysis, and the British Association's annual meeting held a worried debate about psychoanalysis in 1922. Psychoanalysts themselves were worried – If medically qualified analysts referred patients to lay colleagues, could the GMC accuse them of malpractice? (It is illegal for anyone in Britain to practise medicine who is not a qualified medical practitioner.) The National Council for Mental Hygiene proposed to investigate psychoanalysis, but Jones arranged for protests to be made to the medical establishment that 'a lay organization was not the appropriate body to investigate the activities of the medical profession' (King and Steiner, 1991: 12). The BMA accordingly set up its own Committee of Inquiry, which met between 1927 and 1929.

The committee at first included no psychoanalysts, but Jones had himself appointed, and came to dominate it. It began by collecting evidence as to how many medical psychologists (who would now be called psychiatrists) were actually using psychotherapeutic methods. It found that sixty-seven out of seventy-eight did, having begun during or after the war, but that they were very eclectic – most used a mixture of methods, and only twenty-seven had had any Freudian analysis. Committee members produced various alarming stories about therapists – that they encouraged children to a precocious interest in sex, for example – which Jones countered by asking for proof that these were trained analysts, thus encouraging the Committee to believe that there were folk devils around, and there was a danger in treatment by untrained hands. He succeeded in persuading the Committee that Freudian analysis was a safe and effective scientific method for treating neurosis, whereas other forms of psychotherapy relied upon suggestion.

The question of lay analysis was raised. Glover submitted a memorandum about the medical suspicion of psychoanalysis. Because official medical bodies had ignored it, the public were now referring themselves directly to analysts, and unless more people were trained (there were only twenty-five psychoanalysts in practice) the public would end up in the hands of quacks. The medical profession should stop 'vacillating between torpid indifference and splenetic suspicion', accept psychoanalysis, and organize lay analysts into 'a recognized body of trained auxiliaries' such as nurses. Glover represented himself and Jones as holding the line for medicine: 'a small band of medical analysts is engaged in maintaining within the psychoanalytic movement the traditions and etiquette of medical science.' He and Jones agreed that referrals should all be made through doctors, and that lay analysts should work under medical supervision. Jones, who wrote the final report, reiterated Freud's argument: the real lay analyst was the medical man who tried to use psychoanalytic methods without being trained (Minutes of the Committee in Jones's papers, deposited in the British Psychoanalytical Society's archives).

The Committee recommended to the BMA that psychoanalysis be recognized as a branch of medical science with a right to self-regulation. In return for lay analysts undertaking to leave diagnosis and referrals to medical practitioners, the BMA recognized the Society's sole right to train psychoanalysts. The disputes between Melanie Klein and Edward Glover, which became increasingly bitter during the 1930s, were partly because of her increased interest in psychotic processes, hitherto seen as the province of psychiatry.

Gradually, the proportion of analysts who were non-medical and/or women grew. Few psychoanalysts doubted their equal competence – indeed, the two main theoretical factions were both led by laywomen, Anna Freud and Melanie Klein – but many feared for the social status of the profession. When discussions were being held on the post-war reorganization of medicine, the President reported to the 1943 AGM that their position was becoming increasingly precarious. It was attracting too few doctors and too many 'well-educated women . . . we already have more unqualified analysts than our position in the medical world justifies' (King and Steiner, 1991: 483–4). The Society was in a dilemma. If it was to approach the NHS with a view to including psychoanalysis within it, a committee made up of doctors 'would provoke less prejudice and animus'. Psychiatry was developing rapidly, and the Society should be involved – but what would happen to the lay members, whom the medical establishment would not accept as equal colleagues? Some were suspicious that they might be seen as second-class analysts, and in the event the Society stayed outside the NHS.

Recently, the boundaries have shifted again. In 1991, the Society decided to stop requiring lay analysts to ask for medical cover for their work, partly because the medical analysts felt that they couldn't carry responsibility for so many patients, many of whom had not been referred through doctors. Around the same time, it was decided to call analysts with PhDs 'doctor', that is, to cease to give medical qualifications a special place. Perhaps these changes were due to the steady rise of lay members, now standing at over half of new entrants, but perhaps also to the steady proliferation of other therapies, with their own public recognition and complex relationship with the medical profession. Whilst orthodox medicine retains higher status and social recognition, the earlier automatic assumption that doctors are more reliable and responsible people, who should therefore regulate lay analysts on behalf of the public, is now weaker. Psychotherapy, now much more familiar to the general public, need no longer try to derive its claims to legitimacy from medicine, which is now seen as having less hegemony for reasons outlined elsewhere in this volume. Just as it has always done, the transference inside the treatment converts the analyst into all sorts of people; but we need the validation of medicine to establish the external respectability of the profession less than we used to.

Psychoanalysts, like other professions, have increasingly been concerned with the implications of entry into Europe. It is feared that harmonization of qualifications may lead either to the demotion of analysts who are not either doctors or clinical psychologists – that is trained within state-recognized and -regulated specialisms which are made their basis for legitimacy – or to the profession being forced to accept analysts qualified under the less lengthy and intensive trainings abroad. In 1993, the Society banded together with a few other psychotherapy bodies to form a Council to establish a professional register of their own; and yet, in compiling it, we are encouraged to cite our qualifications as doctors and clinical psychologists. That is, the profession is still struggling with how much it can continue to exist wholly outside the assessments of the wider society.

POSTSCRIPT

And what happened to Dora, with whom our story began? We rarely know what happens to patients after they end psychoanalytic treatment. But in 1922 Dora consulted Felix Deutsch, another analyst and Freud's own physician. She had been referred to him with various symptoms connected with her ear – tinnitus, deafness, sleepiness, migraine – which seemed to have no organic cause. She began to complain about her family, and Deutsch recognized her story. She was unhappily married, frigid, dissatisfied with her husband and son, and had become excessively clean and houseproud, like her mother. Deutsch, who obviously disliked her, didn't think he could do anything for her – 'a most repulsive hysteric'. But there is another and rather happier glimpse of her. Contract Bridge became hugely popular in Vienna between the two world wars, and after Herr K.'s death Dora joined forces with Frau K. to teach the game, at which she had become expert (Appignanesi and Forrester, 1992: 167; Deutsch, 1957). I think that Freud, if he knew, would have recognized that she had made good use of her old abilities to show and to conceal, to tell and to deceive.

ACKNOWLEDGEMENTS

I am grateful to Jim Obelkevich, Elizabeth Spillius and Isabel Menzies Lyth for their help with this chapter; but, above all, to my son Saul Budd for his help with the word-processing.

REFERENCES

Appignanesi, L. and Forrester, J. (1992) *Freud's Women*, London: Weidenfeld & Nicolson.

Balint, M. (1957) *The Doctor, His Patient and the Illness*, London: Pitman Medical.

Deutsch, F. (1957) 'A Footnote to Freud's Fragment of an Analysis of a Case of Hysteria', *Psychoanalytic Quarterly*, 26: 159–67.

Frame, J. (1980) *Faces in the Water*, London: Women's Press.

Freud, S. (1905) 'Fragment of an Analysis of a Case of Hysteria', in *The Standard Edition of the Complete Psychological Works of Sigmund Freud*, ed. and trans. J. Strachey, Vol. VII, London: Hogarth, 1953.

Freud, S. (1912) 'The Dynamics of Transference', in *The Standard Edition of the Complete Psychological Works of Sigmund Freud*, ed. and trans. J. Strachey, Vol. XII, London: Hogarth, 1958.

Freud, S. (1915) 'Observations on Transference Love', in *The Standard Edition of the Complete Psychological Works of Sigmund Freud*, ed. and trans. J. Strachey, Vol. XII, London: Hogarth, 1958.

Freud, S. (1926) 'The Question of Lay Analysis', in *The Standard Edition of the Complete Psychological Works of Sigmund Freud*, trans. and ed. J. Strachey, Vol. XX, London: Hogarth, 1959.

Halmos, P. (1965) *The Faith of the Counsellors*, London: Constable.

Heimann, P. (1950) 'On Counter-transference', *International Journal of Psychoanalysis*, 31: 81–4.

Jones, E. (1990) *Free Associations*, London: Transaction Publishers.

King, P. and Steiner, R. (eds) (1991) *The Freud–Klein Controversies 1941–45*, London: Routledge.

Kurzweil, E. (1989) *The Freudians. A Comparative Perspective*, New Haven, CT: Yale University Press.

Racker, H. (1953) 'A Contribution to Problems of Counter-transference', *International Journal of Psychoanalysis*, 34: 313–24.

Rieff, P. (1966) *The Triumph of the Therapeutic – the Uses of Faith after Freud*, London: Chatto & Windus.

Winnicott, D.W. (1949) 'Hate in the Counter-transference', *International Journal of Psychoanalysis*, 30: 69–74.

8   Sharing responsibility for patient care

Doctors and complementary practitioners

David Peters

Why might doctors want to work alongside practitioners trained in the unconventional ways of complementary medicine? Conventional medicine – which is usually identified with biomedicine, the medicine of applied biology – has proven very effective with infection, in deficiency diseases, for problems amenable to surgery, acute pain, anaesthesia and life support. Unfortunately, it has made far less impact on the current epidemic diseases of the West. Stress-, environment- and lifestyle-mediated disease, addiction and psychological disorders seem to respond partially if at all. Nor does the biomedical model easily cope with 'undifferentiated disease', the ordinary kind of unwellness that affects all of us some of the time. And the complex though highly significant interaction of learning, behaviour and lifestyle is beyond its ken. Biomedicine gives an impression of concreteness and certainty, a sense that health can be reduced to biologically determinable elements. But day-to-day health care, far from having sure solutions to disease, is actually riven with uncertainties about causes and cures; its lively complexity is fully reflected in the ideas and beliefs people express about their own health problems and revealed in their attitudes to medicine. Not surprisingly it is in primary care, where people manage their own health problems or seek advice from a wide range of professionals, that complementary medicine is making its presence felt.

General practitioners' (GPs') clinical time is mostly spent dealing with acute self-limiting diseases, with chronic or terminal structural disease, and with long-term relapsing disorders, such as asthma or skin problems – dysfunctional conditions, often with a significant 'stress-related' component. Patients' problems with daily living, and their social crises, also take up a significant amount of time (Fry, 1983). Struggling to meet this range of need, GPs, more readily than hospital specialists, would agree that health care is only partly a matter of science, and realize only too well that biomedicine has no 'cures' for ordinary unwellness and distress even though many patients expect doctors to provide them. Given the post-war progress of biomedicine, it is disappointing that there have been almost no significant pharmaceutical advances in the management of common diseases over the past twenty years (Wetherall *et al.*, 1987).

If we are to understand the changes taking place in primary health care, and in particular the position of complementary medicine, we must appreciate how our ways of thinking are shifting in quite fundamental ways. Yet important cornerstones of the developing world-view have not been integrated into the biomedical frame and this contributes to a growing sense of its inadequacy. Amongst them are: an *ecological-evolutionary perspective*, which implies that organism and environment are not separate, but have co-evolved so that the organism itself is dynamically adapted to the world in a way which determines both its form and function; *homoeostasis*, the organism's self-correcting capabilities which can be assisted to provide an internal stimulus for self-healing; and *the mutual influence of psychological and social factors* on this self-regulation. All these are taken too little into account by clinical science, which has focused so intently on established end-stage disease, even though the central nervous system is now known to ramify via chemical receptors and neurotransmitter substances into every cell of the body. Soul and physiology are interdependent, and psycho-social pressures are met by physiological and potentially patho-physiological responses. This emerging view can be called the 'bio-psycho-social model' of medicine (Engels, 1977). The need for such a framework is at least unconsciously acknowledged by doctors, and so 'whole person care' and 'holistic medicine' have become a kind of professional shorthand for good practice in the 1990s. It is also true that for many people the concept of health itself has become a metaphor for wholeness.

Non-conventional approaches to treatment offered by practitioners of complementary medicine have come into their own within this holistic ethos, because they claim to emphasize care in context, mind–body–spirit interconnectedness, and the importance of catalysing homeostatic processes rather than simply confronting established disease. Systems such as traditional Chinese medicine (TCM), Ayurveda and homoeopathy have some attributes of a more holistic approach, and that might be why, despite a lack of research, doctors as well as patients are attracted to them. Doctors' inability to 'cure' most of the problems presented make them at least curious about whether complementary medicine could provide effective (and less potentially harmful) treatments, and a practical way of manipulating the self-regulation process. And many people do report satisfaction with complementary therapies in a wide range of common illness and disease even when conventional practitioners have failed to provide satisfactory treatment (Consumers' Association, 1986). If features of complementary medicine do have a potential to improve management and quality of life for patients with these conditions, then investigating this role certainly ought to be worthwhile.

It is a truism that primary health care involves both 'doing to' and 'being with' patients, and it does seem that the 'doing to' aspects of practice are in transition. How practitioners handle the 'being with' aspects of their work is also changing, for in a post-paternalistic culture the doctor–patient relationship is bound to change. For some practitioners as well as patients, complementary medicine's appeal may be as another way of constructing the clinical transaction. Patients tell us they want to be seen as whole people, so complementary medicine may be an expression of allegiance to an emergent cultural vision of the person as mind–body–spirit. Patients, sensing complementary practitioners' (CPs') allegiance to this world-view, may find their approach and advice more congruent with their own health beliefs than a doctor's biomedically biased offerings. The all-pervasiveness of the biomedical paradigm, and its relatively unsustaining image of humanity, explain why a return to more traditional values of health care has become so compelling. However, complementary medicine, whether or not it *can* encourage homoeostasis – through its as yet unexplained inter-ventions, or by providing the healing stimuli of time, touch and sense of integration that biomedicine so often lacks – has so far not been shown (even to the most open-minded of the medical establishment) to cure acute, chronic or life-threatening diseases. And biomedicine can often palliate in serious disease where complementary medicine would fail.

So what *can* a GP reasonably expect of complementary medicine? It has been proposed that the integration of complementary practitioners into the NHS could make available an appropriate resource for dealing with func-tional disorders, undifferentiated disease and patients with problems of daily living. Richard Tonkin, while President of the Research Council for Complementary Medicine, wrote

> The long-term benefits that can be expected from successful integration of properly trained and registered complementary therapists with con-ventional scientific practitioners are far reaching. First it would relieve the severely restrictive and indeed often crippling overload with which both the GP and hospital services are faced today. Secondly, it should effect substantial economies in the management of the majority of patients suffering from non-life threatening undifferentiated illness, for whom neither expensive high technology services nor costly and poten-tially toxic agents are necessarily appropriate. In turn this would render these same services more readily available for the minority of patients suffering from specific disease entities for which these same services and medications are unquestionably essential. . . . I would even go so far

as to suggest that a reciprocal partnership between conventionally trained doctors and properly trained complementary practitioners could go a long way towards transforming our existing National Disease Service into a National Health Service in actuality as well as name.

(Tonkin, 1987: 361)

Yet patients consulting CPs not based in general practice can cause significant difficulties for their GPs. Continuity of care, clinical responsibility and GPs' uncertainty about CPs' knowledge, skills and professionalism may become difficult issues (Murray and Shepherd, 1988). It may be that where complementary medicine is split off from general practice, the use of alternative treatment by patients does not lead to an equivalent reduction in demand on general practitioners' time. However, the experience of the group of CPs and GPs with whom I work in an NHS primary care team tends to confirm Richard Tonkin's proposal that collaboration is practical and appropriate within the NHS. According to several surveys, CPs in the private sector are generally consulted by patients with pain and intermittent chronic dysfunction, as well as some clients needing long-term support. Our extended NHS primary care team gets a similar spectrum of clients referred by the practice's GPs.

The CPs – two massage practitioners, an osteopath, a homoeopath and a TCM practitioner – work only two or three half-day sessions each week. The practice also has a social worker/psychotherapist who works as a counsellor for three days a week, and a half-time outreach social worker seeing homeless families in the community. Regular evening classes are held to introduce patients to relaxation skills. The practice, which is in Central London, works alongside a church initiative, one of whose aims is to develop a locally based counselling service, and the pastoral centre and health centre intend to find other ways of co-operating to provide better care in the community. An inner-city setting, a rapidly changing financial climate and the unpredictability of health care provision all ensure that the practice has to prioritize its own use of resources, so the innovative work with CPs is not seen as its raison d'être.

The issues which will determine whether complementary medicine becomes more widely available within the NHS are not simply about proof of efficacy. The question of cost-benefit and how best to manage the resource created by a CP–GP interface will be equally important. To ensure consistently efficient use of their services, we have worked hard to develop adequate referral criteria and agree working practices. However, these are being pushed to their limits as our patient numbers increase and, despite the Department of Health's 1991 ruling that GPs are free to employ CPs, it is increasingly difficult in a cash-limited NHS to find funding for the CP time needed. Although in the private sector patients can, providing they have the fees, refer themselves to CPs ad lib, our patients do not have open access to CPs. Many conventional specialists – who in the United Kingdom expect only to see patients at the request of their GP – would consider it un-professional behaviour to do so without the GP's full approval. So while an open access arrangement might be appropriate in a consumer-centred model of health care, the British convention makes GPs the gatekeeper to many NHS resources. In our centre GPs maintain this role; our attempt to model a new kind of collaboration applicable elsewhere in the NHS would have been marginalized had we done otherwise. Yet the GP's powerful position as controller of patient movement seems to reiterate a historical stereotype of powerful 'establishment' and subordinate 'fringe', so it *could* perpetuate conflict. Still there is much to recommend GPs retaining their role as 'gatekeepers' in the case of complementary medicine, if non-conventional therapies are to become an integral part of mainstream health care. And in countries where GPs do not retain this role – where patients, as in the United States, freely refer themselves to specialists – it seems not only that without a generalist's overview the patient's care becomes frag-mented, but, moreover, that the overall cost of health care rises. Whatever the structure of an NHS incorporating complementary medicine, it is likely that the historical, positional and 'expert' power of doctors will remain, even though few doctors have much more than a layperson's understanding of alternative medical systems such as homoeopathy or TCM.

But if it is the GP's task to refer selectively to CPs, then what criteria can be established? With so slim a grasp of a CP's frame of reference, knowledge-base or skills, it will none the less be doctors who have the authority to make complementary medicine more or less widely accessible within the NHS. So it will be important for future development of colla-boration within the NHS that appropriate learning programmes be available to give GPs a broader understanding of the implications and potential of holistic approaches to health care, including an appreciation of comple-mentary medicine's role. While courses aiming to give GPs an overview of complementary medicine and its place in primary care are gradually becoming available, and are sometimes subsidized by the Department of Health, it is significant that they are generally led by doctors; notably few are as yet organized by non-medical CPs.

Though teamwork is fraught with problems, it seems certain that holistic health care, precisely because the range of knowledge skills and attitudes needed goes so far beyond the purely biomedical, will have to be provided by multidisciplinary teams (BHMA, 1991). In the NHS, many primary care teams already include medical, nursing and social work personnel, who work together across the boundaries of their individual disciplines, and who have to be critically open to a broad range of interventions and health maintenance approaches. How feasible is it then to bring CPs into these teams? Their models of therapeutics are so different from one another's and from GPs' that the similarities between their values, the challenges they face and their prac- tical aims may easily be missed. In our group we have the opportunity at weekly meetings to hold seminars where members can learn about one another's approaches. A fundamental misunderstanding that our group has only recently begun to articulate arises because CPs believe GPs are biomedics, while GPs believe CPs to be specialists. Yet the overlap between their approaches is substantial – therapeutics notwithstanding.

General practice in the United Kingdom has bred a quite special species of generalist, partly because the nature of British family medicine has been so much shaped by patients' 'free' access, and by their very long-term contact with the same GPs, who are able to develop an intimate knowledge of their patients' emotional life, physical body and social predicament. GPs, who know from experience that general practice involves a wide range of therapeutic factors, often make the mistake of seeing comple- mentary medicine as about specialized *technique*, and thus see CPs as specialists rather than as generalists. But is that the case? A specialist focuses on a particular organ system or phase of life and emphasizes cure, whereas the generalist might be consulted over every kind of human problem, and aim to facilitate self-regulation, homoeostasis, prevention and long-term management not only by using treatment but also by offering support and structured self-care. Whereas a specialist focuses on structure and quantity – established pathology – the generalist considers function and quality, bearing in mind the individual's or family's susceptibility, the relevance of triggering factors and levels of resilience. The specialist intervenes definitively in order to produce an outcome; the generalist, while also concerned with cure in those cases where that is feasible, must see this in context and with regard to a multifaceted process of care and containment. Both GP and CP at their best attempt to comprehend how patients' conditions arise out of their individuality, the lives they have led, their relationships and predicaments. This contextual 'diagnosis' may give rise to ideas for ways of encouraging healthy adaptation, promoting recovery or limiting further organic, personal and social damage. Like GPs, CPs facilitate this not only by treatment that gives some symptomatic relief, but also by helping patients develop coping strategies and insight.

The image of a CP as specialist is an obstacle to cooperation, especially if, as Balint (1957) suggests, GPs infantilize themselves by their fantasies of specialists' power to cure. This is a difficult enough dynamic when operating between members of the same professional group, where one of them has a higher level of status and an expertise on which the other may feel dependent. But in a referral between a GP and a hospital consultant at least both parties have some notion of how the other works, having shared a common epistemology and work culture in their training. The psychodynamics of a referral made between professionals who understand very little of one another's health beliefs and working practices will be much more problematic, particularly when doctors already feel vulnerable, alienated by changing patient attitudes, frustrated by medicine's limits, and disappointed by their own struggle with the human condition. The potential for confusion over issues of task, role, credibility, communication and power will then be very great.

If a GP, without understanding clearly what he or she can expect to achieve and why, refers to CPs as if they were 'specialists', then this confers upon CPs a 'magical' status. If, on the other hand, we begin to see CPs as generalists who share many of the primary care team's attitudes to health care, and whose knowledge-base and skills represent a different way of catalysing homoeostasis, then a working relationship becomes possible. Our group has found there are important advantages in reinterpreting CPs as generalists. First, realistic expectations and common achievable aims have followed when we agree to pursue better *management* rather than cure. Second, if we consider that complementary medicine achieves its effects partly by promoting homeostatic processes, then we have the scaffolding for a potential common language. For example, in our clinical conversations we tend to speak about stress and adaptation, to include ideas of mind–body interconnectedness, to incorporate notions of susceptibility/resilience, and to take note of inter- or intra-personal dynamics; ours is a bio-psycho-social language. Third, the primary care team, now less mystified by complementary medicine, has become more able to accept CPs as unthreatening generalists – albeit with different areas of knowledge and skill from a nurse or a doctor – rather than as incomprehensible magical specialists with whom a mainstream health worker has no shared experience.

Michael Balint's (1957) insights into the doctor–patient relationship have been highly influential in the United Kingdom, representing an important strand in GP training, so any serious discussion about the role of complementary medicine in general practice must take his ideas and influence into account. There may be parallels between the way Balint's psychoanalytic ideas have been incorporated into everyday general practice by some GPs, and the growing popularity of non-conventional therapies amongst doctors. Both offer ways forward for practitioners struggling with the challenges of managing difficult patients and the intractable problems associated with chronic disease, psychosomatic, stress-related and functional disorders. Transferential issues abound in the clinical setting and how practitioners work with the relationship is clearly a significant part of the inseparable 'doing' and 'being' that goes on whenever they are with patients. Balint challenged practitioners to become more aware of this aspect of practice, because it made them more effective. Were he alive to do so, he would probably urge CPs as well as GPs to remember that when using a complementary medical approach in clinical 'doing' these issues are no less relevant. However, whereas Balint saw doctors' therapeutic ambition as something to be curbed, CPs, having as yet defined the limits neither of complementary medicine's applicability nor of its effectiveness, appear to retain an air of omnipotence. So, although one might expect the 'listening doctor' to be the most open to complementary medicine, paradoxically there is a potential for profound disagreement between CPs and psycho-dynamically oriented GPs.

Not everyone who comes to a practitioner can be 'fixed'. Many general practitioners, especially those influenced by Balint's psychoanalytic interpretation of GPs' role, see the 'being with' aspects of practice – the 'doctor as drug' – as their main strength. Disputing in particular that primary care is about removing symptoms of 'unorganized illness', for them the GP's task is to accompany patients through ill-health, managing problems that arise and helping contain distress. 'Listening GPs' as well as many CPs realize that patients set great store by a practitioner's 'being with' skills, so there might appear to be considerable common humanistic ground between CPs and GPs. On the other hand, given that CPs are trained to expect to cure their patients, GPs and CPs may easily find themselves polarizing in any debate over 'care' or 'cure'. This has been a core issue for our team, and we have found that a discourse about management of patients rather than their cure avoids inappropriate expectations. If patients can be helped to feel and function better for a time, then we consider a referral from GP to CP justified. We all have needed to examine our emotional attachment to outcome or inappropriate investment in our favoured mode of treatment in order to learn to cooperate. Feelings of omnipotence are a complicating factor (although a powerful therapeutic one at times), and one encouraged for example by homoeopathy's conviction that although its practitioners may fail, its method is infallible. This view is at odds with most GPs', who would observe that any change in chronic disorders is extremely difficult to achieve, and that the realistic strategy means tracking an inexorable course of exacerbation and remission, offering support and limiting damage. A central theme in our CP–GP collaboration has been how to find a middle way between the mania of the former position and the depression of the latter.

It is at least in part this sense of depression and their need to re-examine basic beliefs about health and doctoring that stimulates doctors' curiosity about complementary medicine; it may happen at some transitional point in personal or professional life when a doctor feels uncertain about his or her own power to help. At such a point there might be associated feelings of therapeutic impotence, or burn-out, and even a desire for magical solutions. Perhaps there is a certain sense of omnipotence around the metaphor of health as wholeness, as 'total physical emotional and social well-being' (WHO, n.d.) which resembles biomedicine's implied aim and central myth of extending life and solving all human problems through scientific progress. The wish to have (or to become) a powerful practitioner with the ability to take on all the unbearable, unsolvable problems is understandable; we are compelled by medicine's heroic image, and it is hero myths that challenge us to wrest the prize of cure from the Gods. Few of us – whether doctors or CPs – find it easy to accept that limitation, vulnerability and dependency are also part of being human.

So doctors' interest in complementary medicine may be sparked by a desire to work more 'holistically'; to encourage homoeostasis, and respond appropriately to patients' changing health beliefs. But complementary medicine also appeals as a way of searching for new kinds of 'magic bullets', or of avoiding professional depression. Because several, possibly conflicting, attitudes may be operating simultaneously when CPs and GPs are working together, we have realized the importance of acknowledging them in our team's work. Ambivalence will be around, perpetuating the communication gulf, creating obstacles to sharing clinical management and potentially sabotaging collaboration unless it can be acknowledged and explored.

If complementary medicine's star is currently in the political and clinical ascendant, then it will remain there only if more primary care teams do as ours has and try to integrate CPs. Then the factors which influence cooperation – autonomy and resources, knowledge, language and the complex dynamics of the referral process – can be addressed. If a team works regularly together, the roles of metaphor, congruence, trust, respect – even of positive and negative transference between practitioners – can all be explored, and the whole process of referral, treatment and outcome submitted to the audit cycle. Where doctors and CPs are committed to working together, and discussion time is available, the perspectives of biomedicine, complementary medicine and primary care can all be sympathetically deconstructed, their metaphors explored, shared territory recognized and good boundaries established. Barriers to collaboration begin to fall if this vital time for reflection is allocated. Without it a team is likely to undermine its own work through a lack of clarity about interdisciplinary relationships or unconscious rivalry and professional jealousy. Where there is neither a good enough shared clinical language nor the opportunity to re-align inappropriate expectations by giving feedback, vagueness of diagnosis and a lack of audit into the effect of innovation, plus the tendency to both over- and under-value complementary medicine's role will complete the work of disintegration.

We have found the referral process and the difficulties of inter-disciplinary communication are central problems in CP–GP collaboration, and that they can be gradually worked through as part of the inter-professional development of the extended team. But the time needed for team-building and sharing of ideas and information *is* considerable. Our group feels it needs two hours of meetings a week, even when no joint research project is underway, so that practitioners can share lunch and chat together, discuss ideas about patient management, receive support with problems arising, and explore each other's knowledge-bases, attitudes and beliefs. However, our CPs work at the centre on a part-time basis, so finding the resources in an always busy general practice for over-stretched GPs and CPs to meet regularly has been difficult. If CPs are taking time out from their own private practice, and have accepted a considerable reduc-tion in hourly income in order to establish a foothold in the NHS – with the aim of demonstrating the value of their therapy, and of collaborating with doctors – then opportunities for authentic co-working must be built into any authentically cooperative project.

As well as clinical meetings, we have tried other methods, including sitting in with colleagues (which, though helpful, calls for considerable trust, careful preparation and sensitivity), and videoing consultations, which is less threatening, providing their analysis is properly structured. Accepting a treatment from a colleague may be difficult, but one learns a lot from the experience. Our group also explored the difficulties of colla-boration in a one-year cooperative enquiry (Reason *et al.*, 1992). Two structured joint projects involving all the CPs and GPs have been organized, one aiming at analysing working practices, the other looking into the particular problems arising in a clinic to which patients referred themselves for a consultation with a multidisciplinary group. Both projects incorporated group time where discussion focused on theory and practice related directly to the patients we had seen together, a client-centred approach allowing free exploration of issues in a relatively unthreatening way. Notably, the inclusion of an experienced facilitator in the second project greatly improved the team's ability to make sense of itself, to unravel and describe its own internal processes and manage its work better. We believe the issues revealed – problems of power, resource allocation, differing clinical models, communication and the logistics of the referral process itself – are problematic aspects of CP–GP collaboration. Because they hinder effective collaboration they are relevant to other groups plan-ning similar work (see Reason, 1991), since the seeds of interdisciplinary rivalry may so easily be sown by fantasies of power (the GP's positional, the CP's perceived as unfathomably expert) and privilege (the GP's status and the CP's specialness). Such features of medical– complementary medical cooperation are not unique, but they represent exaggerations, at times bizarre, of typical problems involved in inter- professional and interagency work.

The referral process involves many detailed issues which require collaborative management. A referral to a CP might be made in order to gather information from the practitioner, but given the lack of any common clinical language, and the uneven spread of positional power between doctors and CPs, how might information move between them or joint management be made to work? If the CP is to take over care, then how does that square with GMC regulations about the doctor ultimately carrying responsibility?

When a GP refers out to a CP working elsewhere, the expectations are probably similar to those he or she would have of a conventional specialist; probably 'please fix this' or 'my patient believes you can fix this and has asked to see you'. In-house, a wider exploration of one another's working models and style of work is possible, leading to a more broadly based referral inquiry. Examples from our working together include the following:

What would *your* system call this syndrome/illness/disease?
I think this is a psychosomatic problem, but what do *you* make of it?
Can your therapy offer anything for this patient?
Can your therapy offer anything for this condition?
Have a go and let me know.
I need a break from this patient can you support him/me for a while?
I am curious about your therapy's potential for this patient. Shall we explore together?
I have been treating this patient without much success. Would your approach help?

In our work together we have accepted that a certain pragmatism is inevitable in CP–GP collaboration: in the absence of well-researched referral criteria, all referrals are potentially requests for a trial of treatment. Furthermore, if, as it is said, each complementary medical treatment is individually prescribed, then every treatment becomes an $n = 1$ trial, and this makes selection of suitable cases difficult; the more so if CPs feel a need to impress medical colleagues with good results, in which case even the most challenging referral is unlikely to be refused. But where that is the case poor results will follow.

We have found that the usual factors already influencing referrals include:

1 a patient's wish to see a CP because of his or her own, another's or a reported experience;
2 a GP knowing of a previously successful treatment of a certain type of condition;
3 previously successful treatment of a certain (type of?) patient;
4 a CP's conviction that he or she can successfully treat certain conditions;
5 published or conference reports;
6 a GP's conviction that he or she cannot treat certain conditions (e.g. 'I'm no good with backs');
7 the fact that no conventional treatment options exist/remain/are acceptable;
8 GP's intuition;
9 GP or CP wishful thinking;
10 GP workload or frustration.

GPs in our team have usually referred patients with dysfunctional problems (asthma, migraine, peri-menstrual syndromes, irritable bowel syndrome) and skin problems such as eczema and psoriasis to either the acupuncturist or the homoeopath; back pain and other musculo-skeletal problems to the osteopath. While frankly stress-related dysfunction is less commonly referred, the team's two massage therapists find they see relatively more stress-related somatic complaints than other CPs – and often the very obviously 'unfixable' people. Increasingly, as pressure on their limited time builds up, they find that they can only offer these patients short-term support. Some of these patients are guided towards the practice's relaxation classes (Pietroni, 1992).

Such a common-sense arrangement would be adequate if these conditions were less prevalent, but clearly our small team of CPs can deal with only a small proportion of the patients affected by these common conditions. Informal referral criteria and case review worked at first when patients were fewer and one doctor was working with one CP, but once the team and its workload built up, vague referral criteria became inadequate. Selection of cases could be the key to successful CP–GP teamwork; it is those most likely to benefit who should be referred. Yet in the absence of definitive research to guide us, our group still finds that patients' selection is a continual testing of hypotheses. A therapy's reputation for success with a certain condition or a GPs' recent feelings about 'who treated what well' *is* a fair basis for a referral; but then the learning cycle *must* be completed, and a simple entry into the notes about outcome is inadequate when a great deal of clinical innovation is taking place. Unfortunately, in a busy practice even the necessary brief meetings between several CPs and GPs to review the appropriateness of referrals made, cases in progress and some assessment of their outcome is hard to arrange.

It has taken our team more than six years, and two collaborative inquiry studies grappling with the process issues, to get to the point where we can consider ways of rigorously exploring these referral issues and developing the appropriate data collection procedures. These processes need time, and although 'holistic' settings are rare within the NHS, the practitioners working in them still have to deal with the same pressure of patient demand that most primary care teams face. Time is an issue for demand-led service groups. Yet though it takes time, we have found that our action research can be a lifeline as well as a thread through the maze of CP–GP collaboration, especially where teams have to survive the further internal tensions between supply and demand which are part of the territory in NHS primary care. The process of deciding referral criteria collaboratively and managing them is a real measure of a clinical team's ability to cooperate and make sense of its own working methods. We have achieved a firm grasp of *process* issues, which has been hard-won, and we now have to be equally committed to understanding the *outcome* of our work. However, since our practice serves four thousand patients, adequate feedback is difficult to achieve without a way of integrating clinical data. So we now use computerized data-gathering to tell us which patients are being seen by CPs, why they were referred, to note the 'working complementary medical diagnosis' in use, and therapeutic methods applied. The database also presents an ongoing record of CPs' clinical impressions of progress at each consultation which can be linked to follow-up assessments of outcome (Peters *et al.*, 1994).

Typical problems arise in the process of referral. We have recognized some in our own work, and identified reasons for them. The absence of any referrals might for instance indicate 'I don't understand what you do', 'I don't believe what you claim', 'I don't recognize the need for your contribution' or 'I don't trust you'. Too many could signal 'I don't understand what you do', though they might also indicate 'I am trying to discover your limits', or 'I can't deal with patients with x, y, z. I hope you can'. It could also suggest the organization or individual GP is overstrained or that for some other reason GPs are not 'gatekeeping' adequately. Impossible referrals are sometimes made; not always unwittingly: perhaps when a GP feels disempowered, de-skilled, passive/aggressive, or over-optimistic. Obviously if opportunities for adequate feed-back from CP to GP are not in place, inefficient use of a CP resource and inappropriate expectations will be perpetuated.

Even where an extended team is available, 'fat envelope' patients still confound practitioners' attempts to cure them, and there will inevitably be some patients who move from one CP to another, taking up a disproportionate share of a health care resource which, even expanded to include CPs, is still inevitably a limited one. Several types of multiple consulter can be recognized. The *consumer* is keen to shop around and get the most out of the system, while the *desperate mechanic* believes there must be an externalizable solution to his condition/distress. This patient is searching for the external intervention that will fix him, and because of complementary medicine's pragmatism, its air of omnipotence and the 'have a go factor' a CP may be tempted to rise to the challenge even in circumstances where therapeutic ambition would be better tempered with caution. The *heartsink patient* will always feel the latest practitioner is not good enough, or feel compelled to compare available practitioners to an idealized figure who once made her better. On encountering such patients, as one senses that their problems are overwhelming (for them as well as for you) and that one will not be a good enough practitioner, one's heart sinks. These patients always have thick files of notes, having previously been referred to every available resource because either they or their GP was driven to desperation by their problem. It seems that better teamwork, with a jointly agreed management plan and a clear key worker is more likely to contain these patients' distress (see Gerard and Riddell, 1988), and undoubtedly these patients with persistent unorganized illness, who are often chronically depressed or anxious, or with problems of daily living, do need help to become less dependent on multiple consulting. The *iatrogenic multi-consulter*, on the other hand, is a category, possibly overlapping with any of the above, engendered by doctors who repeatedly refer a difficult patient, perhaps under pressure from the patient, perhaps because of their own anxiety or problems of daily doctoring, or because they still hope to find a practitioner or a therapy who, despite evidence to the contrary, will be able to help. Patients like these need to be protected from specialists of whatever ilk, conventional or otherwise, and there is a more than theoretical danger that if complementary medicine were more widely available, they would come to rely inappropriately on regular visits to CPs.

The reason for these difficult exploratory referrals, and a core issue for collaborative research, is to discover whether what appears 'unorganized illness' to a conventional practitioner is in the light of a complementary medical system a recognizable syndrome on which the appropriate CP can exert specific therapeutic leverage. For example, recurrent back pain, to conventional medicine an apparently unorganized condition which is difficult to grapple with, is seemingly well dealt with by chiropractors and osteopaths. Might there be parallels in other systems where CPs recognize distinct syndromes and treat them effectively even though doctors find in them only chaotic signals of distress? Are there patients for whom the 'talking cures' are inappropriate, yet who do well when the therapeutic space is structured along complementary medical lines? Designing studies to test such hypotheses would be challenging. However, whether or not complementary medical approaches in some objectifiable way 'cure' patients of hard to treat health problems, their role in the management of some patients is, in our experience, a helpful one. Primary care devotes much of its time to patients with chronic problems – some do have physical diseases which may be chronic, others suffer with intermittent dysfunction, or problems of daily living. GPs are likely to see CPs as a potential resource for managing such patients, and some of the problems that arise have already been mentioned. In our group, CPs have accepted that part of their work is about long-term management of patients who temporarily need regular appointments with a CP as part of a strategy to help contain chronic distress or pain. In such cases cure is not the aim. The demand for long-term support might focus complementary medicine's application in the NHS on this group of patients. If so, acute cases will be selected out. Once again it seems that only a well-structured approach, minimizing inappropriate referrals and ensuring efficient use of scarce resources, could make time available for a broadly based use of the service.

When our group first came together, time was relatively protected by research funds which pump-primed our study of the centre's innovative approach. Consequently no one questioned whether the time-frame of CP private practice was appropriate. Long appointments – typically thirty to sixty minutes were given. The NHS GPs, meanwhile, were often seeing eight or more patients an hour for up to five or six hours a day and carrying the responsibility for administration and management of the centre as well as undertaking out of hours cover for its patients. Understandably, this differential fuelled conflict about power, responsibility and privilege, and GPs felt at times that such long appointments over-stretched the resources of a busy NHS health centre. Should the practice of complementary medicine adapt itself to a resource-limited, high-demand system, and if so, how? Perhaps there are lessons to be learned from the failure of psychoanalysis to make much impact in the NHS. There are parallels to be drawn between the way complementary medicine might develop in this context and the way brief forms of psychotherapy developed – particularly in the United States – as a response to resource limitation. Is 'brief-intervention'-TCM, -massage, -homoeopathy or -osteopathy, perhaps based on a thirty- or even twenty-minute 'NHS unit', practical or desirable? *Do* CPs need to see patients for forty minutes to an hour at each visit? If so, then few people will be able to consult them unless many sessions are available, waiting lists unacceptably long, or CP pay unacceptably low. Yet time and touch *are* important elements, so could a CP consultation be shorter without fundamental detriment? Our group is testing out solutions to the problem.

Many of the obvious obstructions to collaboration are removed when the primary care team includes CPs – private fees for service, delays in communicating relevant background or clinical findings, logistical problems in sharing management and follow-up. Yet as these barriers come down, not only do CPs run the risk of being swamped, but it also becomes clear that there are more fundamental and less concrete obstacles to authentic cooperation; the lack of a common clinical language being the most significant. Language barriers, and the lack of valid guidelines on referral and professional status, indicate deeper divisions about which Erich Fromm reminds us:

> Man . . . has a vital interest in retaining his frame of orientation. His capacity to act depends upon it and in the last analysis, his sense of identity. If others threaten him with ideas that question his own frame of orientation, he will react to those ideas as if to a vital threat.
>
> (Fromm, 1972)

These challenges are part of the territory for those engaged in any kind of interprofessional work, because

> each profession acts in a sense like a tribe. Members are nurtured in distinctive ways, they develop their concepts in exclusive gatherings (called professional training, or college membership), they have their own leaders and pecking orders. Like all tribal societies they impose sanctions on non-conforming members. If a member takes on the reality constructs of another tribe, then he or she may even be threatened with exclusion.
>
> (Kilcoyne and Pietroni, 1990)

While the language of tissues and organs may well be appropriate when referring a patient with structural disease to a surgeon, a different 'language' is needed when referring a patient with musculo-skeletal dysfunction to an osteopath. Linked to tactile and visual pattern recognition, an osteopath's language of tissue tension patterns might convey little meaning to a practitioner unfamiliar with the 'dialect' (McDonald and Peters, 1986). Yet the 'musculo-skeletal wing' of complementary medicine is, relatively speaking, a sibling to biomedicine, compared to traditional Chinese medicine (TCM), which is barely even a distant cousin. So what information should a referring doctor include in a referral to a TCM practitioner? Understanding of organic dysfunctions like asthma, migraine or irritable bowel syndrome are potentially enriched by the language and conceptual map of Chinese medicine, which, through its depiction of qualities, blurs the boundaries between physical, psychological and environmental factors. The resulting enlivened picture of a psychosomatic illness, by firing the imagination, can help individualize the problem, facilitating empathy, insight and possibly even appropriate therapeutic action (Peters *et al.*, 1993). But how, in feeding back to a referring GP, could an acupuncturist convey this?

When cooperating in patient management or when facilitating any interdisciplinary work, the common language we develop will be crucial, and in the absence of any other our collaborative group adopted a modified bio-psycho-social language. Patrick Pietroni (1991) has described the variety of languages used in health and community care, pointing out that among them is the 'language of energy'. The word 'energy' is often used by practitioners of complementary medicine as though it described something objective. But it is actually metaphorical, implying some substrate through which complementary medicine's homoeostatic interventions might act. It is part of complementary medicine's 'ecology of ideas' to the extent that one can be sure a therapy is complementary medicine-like if it uses the 'energy metaphor'. It also illustrates the sense in which we are searching for a construct capable of authentically underpinning and uniting the disparate complementary therapies. Linking energy to well-being is now part of a vernacular health language; we may lack it; have too much, or an imbalance of it. It is sometimes said to be blocked, or disordered, and we all know what it feels like 'to have too little'. Yet for a medical practitioner with a conventional scientific training, 'energy' also evokes images of Newtonian billiard ball mechanics, or the biochemical pathways of carbohydrate metabolism. Although it is fashionable to speak of our living post-Einstein, and to remind ourselves that most matter is empty space bound up with 'energy', most people remain as mystified by the quantum model as they are by theological concepts of 'energy' as the relativistic ground of being. Unfashionable though it may be to question whether the same 'energy' is the object of both descriptions of reality, it seems in any practical sense that 'energy' was a construct already too thinly stretched even before it gained currency as the basis of health, and health itself mutated into a metaphor about personal integration.

The language of medical training is scientific reductionism, which aims at being *rigorous*. Complementary medicine systems tend to adopt more qualitative, process-oriented descriptions of the body; they are potentially more systemic and dynamic in their approach and less preoccupied with structure. They aim to be more *relevant* to human experience. The biomedical is fundamentally unlike any complementary medicine model, and this difference raises interpersonal and interdisciplinary issues not unlike the undercurrents besetting relationships between men and women. Here, too, despite the undeniable potential one might have for complementing the other, a sense of otherness incites polarization and separateness. The dynamics of working relationships between doctors and CPs are easily distorted by basic differences between their clinical concepts. However, primary care is not synonymous with biomedicine, and although GPs and CPs groping for more holistic diagnosis and treatment may agree to constrain their discussions within a bio-psycho-social or psycho-dynamic framework, practitioners may still find themselves in an unexpected struggle for dominance when their viewpoints seem irreconcilable. Clearly the psycho-dynamic frame, inasmuch as it fails to address either the interdependency of mind, body and spirit or the nature of health, is a poor substitute for real common ground. So, as often as not, 'energy' – a wild card whose face value any player may name, but which leaves everyone guessing as to the rules of the construct game being played – is used as if it were an explanation.

Any working group aiming at synthesis will have to question and transcend the limitations inherent in the languages and beliefs of its constituent professional tribes. The example of 'energy' is only one of the clichés needing to be subverted. 'Energy' is said to be at work in social and emotional, spiritual and physical aspects of life. And obviously it is. But some differentiation of qualities must be possible, and indeed some Eastern systems – TCM and Ayurveda – as well as the European synthesis known as anthroposophical medicine do attempt it. A scientist would find all this talk of 'energy', and the wooliness of thought that often accompanies it, alienating, a dismissive insult to the splendidly differentiated intellectual construct of science. But insofar as the 'energy metaphor' hints at some sort of shared subjectivity, it takes on a sacramental quality, hinting as it does at all we do not fully understand about the mind–body–spirit–environment relationship, and dimly perceived organizing principles at work. 'Energy' is a mystery word and perhaps, once the term *has* been deconstructed and accepted as abstract and subjective, it can be used as such in a working group. Still, a group trying to develop a common clinical language may find, as ours has, that careless use of the energy metaphor is a source of confusion; a noun which obstructs the search for necessary adjectives. For the sake of its own development, our interprofessional group had to confront such mystification, and risk desecrating a comfortably shared but unexamined energy myth. The process of exploring one's own and others' subjectivity is not always comfortable; even less so where pet beliefs have to be overthrown.

So a core problem for complementary practitioners and for collaboration with biomedics is that neither a common language, nor a solution to the related need for a unified approach to all that the 'energy metaphor' stands for is yet available. However, in a group reflecting on patients, our practitioners still found that some of the time they could share their different subjective impressions and interpretations of clinical phenomena, and confront the problems of communication and the challenges of joint decision-making. CP–doctor working groups are an intense microcosm of a culture struggling with an emergent paradigm and they probably generate even more difficult dynamics than other interdisciplinary working groups. So it is understandable that the tone and content of the BMA's (1986) first report on alternative medicine (as the British Holistic Medical Association's response to it illustrated [BHMA, 1986]) implied that the very existence of alternative systems of medicine represented a challenge of heretical dimensions. It is particularly this aspect of complementary medicine, its counter-cultural nature, that makes the problems of collaboration so particularly potent and focused. Consequently the process of mapping the unconscious, conceptual and organizational turbulence collaboration creates means having to excavate the foundations of our own health beliefs, how we construct them, and what the phenomenal rise of complementary medicine has to tell us about emerging constructs of reality. Our culture has been profoundly intertwined with the values and beliefs of biomedicine, and if, as some authors have suggested (see, e.g., Capra, 1982) the rise of complementary medicine is part of a wider cultural upheaval, then we can expect that where the languages of new and old health care sub-cultures collide there will be conflict. The discourse about health is inevitably about human nature itself, and the validity of developing new metaphors or different languages in health care raises issues of paradigm power.

> Clinicians from different disciplines clash because while they may agree about what the patient needs, they interpret those needs through different frameworks, and bring to the situation fundamentally different assumptions about what an intervention may do. . . . Beyond the interpersonal disagreements and the structural differences, something else is around (although these superficial conflicts will multiply the effects of the deeper ones). People will suddenly find themselves in conflict they did not expect. They will not be able to express themselves in words clearly. They will feel their world is taken over. I think this might well be called paradigmatic power struggle.
>
> (Reason, 1991)

The more recent BMA pronouncements on the possible usefulness of complementary medicine suggest that the floodgates of patient demand for complementary medicine in the NHS may be about to open. Issues of registration, professional indemnity and discipline are identified in the BMA's new report (1993), which acknowledges not only that public demand has grown beyond the point where the BMA can adopt an ivory-tower attitude to developments, but also that CP training and professionalization have raced ahead in the seven years since the Association's first ill-informed attempt to grapple with complementary medicine. In the opinion of this new report, it is research into the validity of non-conventional therapies that will determine its place in the NHS. But the wide array of influences outlined in this chapter illustrate how complex collaboration between doctors and CPs is likely to be, and in the highly competitive struggle for research grants it may be that these factors will make it even more difficult to gain credibility and funding for research into complementary medicine. Unfortunately the Department of Health has so far been unwilling to ringfence money for this important R & D.

Practitioners' unconscious beliefs are significant aspects of the intellectual and emotional investment they make in their work as practitioners; important features of attachment to their clinical world-view. By making us partisan in our allegiance to certain approaches, they exemplify one kind of sensitive area potential collaborators may feel they need to protect. As in any team, professional pride will sometimes be seen as arrogance or provoke confrontation. For example, in one joint consultation a doctor who had studied homoeopathy and an acupuncturist were talking about a patient with high blood pressure in the lungs caused by a structural chest disease. When the acupuncturist, a senior practitioner with an extensive grounding in psychotherapy, began to talk about the possibility that Chinese medicine could influence this structural circulatory disorder, the doctor expressed disbelief and ill-concealed scorn. His complementary medicine colleague, incensed by this reaction, accused the doctor of intellectual arrogance. The doctor paused, surprised by the vigour of his own response, only grudgingly accepting that he had no definite basis for refuting the acupuncturist's assertion. Even if he had, the confrontational style learned on many hospital teaching rounds, where it might have passed unnoticed in the clash of ideas between two medics, was an inappropriate and somehow shocking way of transacting a clinical discussion with a peer clinician from a different 'tribe'.

What had been revealed was an unconscious lack of respect for another's world-view. The ensuing argument and the practitioners' eventual reconciliation over a period of several months of working together, was reminiscent of a clash between disciples of opposing religions who, having recognized the potential for harm implicit in their irreconcilable positions, struggle to find a way of co-existing and so grow into an authentic regard for one another. This is no easy journey, but it is a way that has to be travelled if we are to explore the sometimes confused subject–object relations that all clinical work, but especially collaborative work across systems of medicine, throws up.

Without close working relationships, dialogue between complementary medicine and the mainstream becomes difficult because of two commonly witnessed attitudes. The first position, denial of the conflict, has contributed to the creation of an autonomous complementary medicine sub-culture which pays lip service to the idea that complementary medicine and biomedicine complement one another but avoids exploring how, when or why. Second, and worse, is the projection of blame – for the failure of biomedicine's theory and practice or for the folly of its practitioners – on to conventional medicine. This has produced anti-medical elements in complementary medicine's sub-culture which would deny biomedicine any relevance whatever.

Tension between one's individual and group nature is part of the human psychic territory; we are simultaneously fascinated and appalled by similarities and differences. Consequently the third way, towards co-existence with the powerful forces of conventional health care, will remain by far the most difficult route for doctors and CPs to take, and it may prove impossible unless clinical pluralism can be validated. Controlled clinical trials alone, however, will not facilitate cooperation, and close collaboration between doctors and complementary practitioners – stimulating and clinically innovative though it can be – will continue to be the exception unless more doctors and CPs in attempting to work side by side can not only find the resources to do so and learn to tolerate the difficulties, but also explore the important meaning behind the discomfort, uncertainty and anxiety that working together will sometimes engender. It will be worth the effort.

ACKNOWLEDGEMENT

I would like to acknowledge the inspirational part played by Patrick Pietroni in creating and maintaining Marylebone Health Centre, and my thanks for his support and participation in our groping for understanding. Grateful thanks go to all my all colleagues there, and especially to Patrick, Arnold Desser and Peter Davies, for exploring with me the ideas that this chapter tries to express. My thanks also go to Peter Reason, whose heroic spirit of inquiry struck a spark that still enlivens our CP–GP collaboration.

REFERENCES

Balint, M. (1957) *The Doctor, His Patient and the Illness*, London: Pitman Medical.
BHMA (1986) *BHMA Response to the BMA's Report: Alternative Therapy*, London: BHMA.
BHMA (1991) *Response to the Department of Health's Green Paper 'The Health of the Nation'*, London: BHMA.
BMA (1986) *Alternative Therapy: Report of the Board of Science and Education*, London: BMA.

BMA (1993) *Complementary Medicine: New Approaches to Good Practice*, Oxford: Oxford University Press.

Capra, F. (1982) 'The Biomedical Model', in *The Turning Point*, Aldershot: Wildwood House.

Consumers' Association (1986) 'Magic or Medicine?', *Which?*, October: 443–8.

Engels, G. (1977) 'The Need for a New Medical Model: The Challenge for Biomedicine', *Science*, 4286: 129–35.

Fromm, E. (1972) *The Anatomy of Human Destructiveness*, London: Jonathan Cape.

Fry, J. (1983) *Common Diseases, Their Nature, Incidence and Care*, Lancaster and Boston, MA: MTP Press.

Gerard, T.J. and Riddell, J.D. (1988) 'Difficult Patients: Black Holes and Secrets', *British Medical Journal*, 297: 530–2.

Kilcoyne, A. and Pietroni, P.C. (1990) 'The History of the Primary Care Team', in *RGCP Yearbook*, London: RGCP.

McDonald, R. and Peters, D. (1986) 'Osteopathy', *Practitioner*, 230: 1073–8.

Murray, J. and Shepherd, S. (1988) 'Alternative or Additional Medicine? A New Dilemma for Doctors', *Journal of the Royal College of General Practitioners*, 38: 511–14.

Peters, D., Desser, A., Jago, W. and McEwen, L.M. (1993) 'Irritable Bowel Syndrome', *Complementary Therapies in Medicine*, 1: 14–18.

Peters, D., Davies, P. and Pietroni, P. (1994) 'Introducing osteopathy to general practice: an audit cycle', London: NW Thames AHA.

Pietroni, P. (1991) 'Towards Reflective Practice – The Languages of Health and Social Care', *Journal of Interprofessional Care*, 6(3): 7–16.

Pietroni, P. (1992) 'Beyond the Boundaries – The Relationship between General Practice and Complementary Medicine', *British Medical Journal*, 305: 564–6.

Reason, P. (1991) 'Power and Conflict in Multidisciplinary Collaboration', *Journal of Complementary Medical Research*, 5(3): 144–50.

Reason, P., Chase, H.D., Desser, A., Melhuish, C., Morrison, M., Peters, D., Wallstein, D., Webber, V. and Pietroni, P. (1992) 'Towards a Clinical Framework for Collaboration between General and Complementary Practitioners', *Journal of the Royal Society of Medicine*, 85: 161–4.

Tonkin, R.D. (1987) 'Role of Research in the Rapprochement between Conventional Medicine and Complementary Therapies: Discussion Paper', *Journal of the Royal Society of Medicine*, 80: 361–3.

Wetherall, D.J., Ledingham, J.G.G. and Worrell, D.A. (1987) 'Preface', in *Oxford Textbook of Medicine*, Oxford: Oxford University Press.

WHO (n.d.) *The Alma Ata Declaration*, Geneva: WHO.

9 'Only nature heals'

A discussion of therapeutic responsibility from a naturopathic point of view

Richenda Power

There are aspects of therapeutic responsibility peculiar to naturopathic practice. Some of these will be identified and discussed with reference to the philosophical bases of 'nature cure', recently better described as 'nature care' (Muirhead, 1992). Some will be discussed with regard to specific dilemmas arising from practice. First, a brief outline of naturopathy is given for the reader who may be unfamiliar with the practice.

Naturopathy is the professional practice of 'nature cure', historically a collection of methods and abstinences thought to enable a person to move toward 'high level health' (J. Thomson, n.d.; see C.L. Thomson, 1966). Nature cure can consist of positive inputs, such as mineral- and vitamin-rich nutrition, stimulation or relaxation through the use of water (bathing, splashing, paddling, compressing and packing), exercise; and abstinences, for example occasional fasting and complete rest. There are situations where it may be more therapeutic to remove oneself from an intolerable situation, whether at work or in a relationship, than to rely on propping oneself up (say with 'uppers' like tea, coffee or other stimulants, or 'downers' like alcohol or valium). There are also situations where using methods such as stress management and assertion, or simply taking breaks, can enable one to survive in a healthier way. Anyone may put 'nature cure' into effect in their own life, without necessarily ever consulting a professional practitioner. Most of us manage to obey 'nature's laws' to some extent anyway, without reference to any printed instructions: we feed ourselves, are active, breathe, wash and get some rest and sleep.

'Nature cure' as professional health care advice has sometimes been belittled as 'lifestyle' medicine supreme, an approach often criticized as one that might 'blame the victim' for their illness, without always taking account of the constraints on our lives such as poverty, poor housing, work demands or unemployment (e.g. Crawford, 1980). In the West the professional history of 'nature cure' in the nineteenth and early twentieth century tended to be one of doctors 'seeing the light' and ceasing to prescribe from their existing pharmacopoeia (Power, 1984, 1989; Twigg, 1982). Thenceforward they advocated the use of fasting, 'food reform' (e.g. the use of whole cereals, fruit and vegetables, and often vegetarianism), dress reform, methods of bathing in air, sunlight and water, exercises, rest and methods of mental relaxation. Some of these doctors became well-known heads of sanatoria (e.g. Dr Lindlahr); some were struck off their professional registers for teaching the public about health (e.g. Dr Allinson, Sir Arbuthnot Lane). Professional training outside medicine appears to have become available primarily through sanatoria in the United States and some areas in Europe. The first training available full-time in Britain was at the Edinburgh School of Natural Therapeutics (ESNT), established shortly after the First World War by James Thomson, who himself had studied at several sanatoria in the United States. Various part-time and correspondence courses were also available from around that time in Britain, one of which eventually developed (by the mid 1960s) into a full-time four-year course offered by the British College of Naturopathy and Osteopathy (BCNO), London, which is currently the only full-time undergraduate course available in the country. The situation in the various states of North America, in Canada and in Germany is rather different, with a majority of naturopaths having studied medicine first before specializing in what is now often called 'naturopathic medicine'.

There are significant philosophical differences between the treatment/modality-inclined naturopath and the opposite pole, which the ESNT graduates would refer to as the 'straight nature cure practitioner'. (Chiropractors similarly use the words 'straights' and 'mixers' to distinguish between the purists and the more eclectically inclined practitioners (Power, 1984.) No doubt similar divisions exist between individual naturopaths' outlooks even where they have all emerged from the same school, and it should not be thought that the practitioners produced by any one would necessarily hold identical positions. The significance of this split is mainly to do with the place of 'remedies' or 'adjuncts' in naturopathic practice.

The 'straight nature cure practitioner' and their even purer cousins, the 'natural hygienists' (see Roth and Hanson, 1976), eschew the use of any form of 'remedy', whether it be a vitamin supplement, a homoeopathic pill or an antibiotic.[1] At root this is because it is held that 'only nature heals', a saying that is the motto for the British Naturopathic Association (BNA), although both 'straights' and 'mixers' would be found among its members. The Incorporated Society of Registered Naturopaths (ISRN) maintains a 'straight' stance in only accepting for membership those naturopaths who forswear the use of any 'remedies'. This is because it is thought that their use might encourage a dependence by the patient on the remedy itself, rather than the healing power of nature. Tied up with such a notion is a philosophical debate about the idea of 'cure'. James Thomson, the pioneer naturopath in Britain, used to say,

> A man [*sic*] may no more partake of a cure that will cure him for the rest of his life than he may take a bath that will keep him clean for the rest of his life. Any cure that is worthwhile has to be worked at.

(n.d.: 8)

This chapter is written by a practising naturopath whose first contact with 'nature cure' was as a patient herself over twenty years ago. She consulted a graduate of the Edinburgh school so her first framework for understanding naturopathy was 'straight' although her later professional training was at the more eclectic British College of Naturopathy and Osteopathy. On graduation from that course she applied for membership of the ISRN and was happy to forswear the use of 'remedies'. The main part of the discussion that follows has been shared with colleagues from that membership, but represents only her own views as a practitioner of the 'straight' variety. Because of this I have chosen to write in the first person when I am speaking for myself, reverting to an impersonal style when describing such matters as ethical codes of professional societies or historical situations.

It is often difficult to write about 'nature cure' without automatically resorting to the use of a mythologized and stereotypical model of medical practice for comparative purposes. I want to try to avoid this essentially negative method of reactive criticism and to aim to build a positive model of naturopathic practice with which to discuss therapeutic responsibility. To do this I shall describe the practitioners' view of their position, and their view of their relationship with the patient and the healing process, and all of these within the wider society. This is because I believe that naturopathy has a wholesome and positive contribution to make to debates on health care and therapeutic responsibility in its own right, and an appreciation of this can sometimes be weakened by the use of a stereotypical, homogeneous and monolithic view of a 'body of knowledge' called medicine.

THERAPEUTIC RESPONSIBILITY

Considering issues of therapeutic responsibility makes one review a wide range of central naturopathic concepts. 'Only nature heals' has been a central tenet of naturopathic philosophy, but it could equally be applied across the board to all healing, whether the person experiencing healing is 'looking after themselves' or is in the care of, for example, doctors, spiritual healers, nurses, friends or naturopaths. Whatever agency is involved, at the bottom line of analysis, only if the patient's 'healing ability'[2] or 'vitality' is present, which is a natural capacity, will healing occur. We can think of the 'vitality' as a composite of genetic endowment, a functioning physiology, psychology and spiritual 'will to live' if you like.

To state this is not to let practitioners 'off the hook' in terms of therapeutic responsibility. Jill Rakusen has pointed out that the concept of nature's healing can be abused by some practitioners so that the slow-to-heal, or non-healing, patient may be blamed for not following instructions:

> While alternative practitioners are well in advance of conventional medicine in appreciating the subtleties involved in health and disease, they have a long way to go before they can be considered truly holistic (i.e. incorporating social and political awareness into their practice). All too easily, they can end up 'blaming the victim', oblivious to the many ways in which our oppressive society affects us.
>
> (1989: 102)

Sometimes, she argued, a therapist could use

> a cast iron let-out which leaves their reputation intact if we remain ill: far from questioning the appropriateness of their own approach, some are far too ready to off-load any responsibility for the situation, claiming or suggesting, for example, that 'You haven't tried hard enough'.
>
> (1989: 102)

She termed this the 'Heads I win, tails you lose' phenomenon, implying that practitioners should examine their consciences and improve their accountability. Straight nature cure may well have an advantage over many other systems here in the concept of the 'healing crisis', which re-defines illness as the body's attempt to heal. 'Remain[ing] ill' need not be viewed negatively, but as practitioners we would be committed to trying to understand what the whole situation was about, and to sharing that thinking with the patient together with our concern for their comfort and future healing.

The patient usually comes to the naturopath by choice. A few people in Britain may now have access to naturopaths via their general practitioners on the National Health Service and therefore may have been referred, rather than choosing a practitioner themselves. At the time of writing this is rare. The patient who has chosen the practitioner expects something from the interaction, and is usually paying for the consultation. Practitioners have set themselves up as professionals, experts with specialist knowledge. (See Power, 1989 for a discussion of the paradoxes involved in claiming specialist knowledge in 'the natural'.) There is the concept of some sort of contract involved between patient and practitioner and it is that which we are to look at here. It could be called 'a healing bond', as the editors of this volume suggest, but, interestingly, the word 'bond' is used both for contracts and for close connections, psychological, emotional and/or physical, between people. I would like to consider both these aspects (there may be more): the contract[3] and the relationship.

A contract

Let us start with the idea of the contract. There are expectations not only on the patient's side in nature cure, but also on the practitioner's. As naturopaths we make it our business quite quickly from the beginning of our first consultation to start a process of definition or re-definition of what healing is: often a re-education of ideas about health and illness. Expectations from patient and practitioner confront each other, shifting and changing during our first hour of meeting. We try to get across the ideas that 'only nature heals', that the body is an intelligent organism with self-healing powers. Such opportunities often arise spontaneously in answer to the patient's questions: 'Can you cure me?', or very often over the telephone 'Can you cure condition x?' We share our conviction that if we could carefully review the patient's life history (with an emphasis on healing events rather than disease events) we would together begin to understand the process which has brought the patient to us today. We emphasize that we are therapeutically interested in causes rather than symptoms.

At the same time the patient's primary reason for being with us must be respected. We must not forget that this is what has motivated them to come to us for help. Whilst explaining that we never offer cure, we nevertheless offer 'nature care', thereby enabling healing to occur naturally. But it is our very expertise, our understanding and interpretation of 'nature's ways' or 'laws' that enable us to offer, in James Thomson's phrase, 'the intelligent leaving alone'. I personally do not like the adjective 'intelligent' because it implies that other 'leaving alone' is stupid, whereas what he meant was informed or trained.[4] What the phrase means in practice is not rushing in, for example, to suppress fever or spots in every case, but welcoming their advent often as the body's intelligent attempt to self-heal. I think the choice of phrase 'intelligent leaving alone' has to be seen in its historical context also. In the nineteenth century there was some movement among doctors to 'laissez-faire' where it was felt that nothing either therapeutically useful or perhaps economically wise (particularly with poor patients, or those whom the medic may have deemed better not alive to breed) should be done. Such a 'leaving alone' was not what James Thomson intended. With him, as with Lindlahr, it was the practitioner's experience, expertise and diagnostic skills that should enable a full assessment of the patient's vitality, and whether they were undergoing a 'healing crisis' (the body's self-healing event) or a 'disease crisis' (a sign of degeneration and lack of vitality). Often the acute 'healing crisis' is best left alone and interference, whether allopathic, homoeopathic, herbal or whatever, may only prove a hindrance to the body's intentions. This applies equally well to emotional crises: for example grief, as a human response to loss, is usually best allowed to happen rather than to be chemically or emotionally suppressed or denied.

To know when to 'leave alone' and when not is critical to good and safe practice. So also is knowing when to refer, and to whom. We can acknowledge that part of the contractual aspect of our therapeutic responsibility as naturopaths is our training, both academic and practical, our information, our ongoing knowledge-base and its application. This is a matter not just for the individual but is the subject of agreement by the profession as a whole.

I would like to examine a contractual aspect of group responsibility here by looking at ethical codes. The *Bye-Laws of the Incorporated Society of Registered Naturopaths* (1990) have a section on 'Professional Conduct'. It reads as follows:

14. (a) *Methods*: No Member of the Register shall prescribe 'remedies', e.g., biochemicals, tissue salts, hormones, vitamin concentrates, pharmaceutical, homoeopathic or herbal preparations; neither shall he [*sic*] practise hypnotism or any other therapy contrary to the philosophy and principles of the Society.

(b) *Titles and Initials*: A Member may describe himself [*sic*] as 'Registered Naturopath', as 'on the British Register of Naturopaths' or as 'Member of the Incorporated Society of Registered Naturopaths', as appropriate, but shall not use the initials of these bodies so as to suggest the possession of a degree. Members are recommended to use no initials after their names other than those of degrees they have received from Universities or State Recognized Colleges.

(c) *Advertising*: Individual advertisements may contain, in addition to name, qualifications, address and telephone number, only mention of Register and/or Society Membership and such information as may be essential to enable the prospective patient to reach the practitioner.

Members shall not, either in advertisement or on stationery, mention diseases treated, apparatus or special modalities used . . .

(d) *Assistants*: Members may employ as assistants persons not on the Register, such as masseurs, remedial gymnasts, physiotherapists, provided that such assistants are:

(i)   effectively supervised, and:

(ii) given specific instructions for each patient.

It is perhaps disappointing that the majority of the above statements are phrased in negative form, but it is understandably easier to write a short list of 'thou shalt nots' than to try to encompass all the positive aspects of good practice. It is possible to tease out some of the underlying intentions that relate to therapeutic responsibility. The issue dealt with under 'Methods' has in part been discussed at the beginning of this chapter, and is to do with the concern not to mislead the patient into looking to anything other than nature as the source of 'cure'. The avoidance of hypnotism maybe takes us further into the issue of therapeutic responsibility, as it is to do with discouraging a dependence by the patient on the practitioner, hypnotism being seen as the control of one person by another.[5] Since the whole drift of nature cure is towards encouraging the individual to enjoy life as it is lived through them uniquely, there can be no place for a controlling force from outside. Where hypnotism ends and relaxation therapy begins is still a hotly debated subject within the ISRN, the finer points of argument turning upon the nature of suggestion.

The details about how members should describe themselves can be appreciated in a historical context of some non-medical practitioners parading bogus degrees (e.g. Littlejohn of the British School of Osteopathy 1931, see Larkin, 1983). The ISRN was formed in 1934 and members were encouraged to have none of this, to be ultra-'professional'. Although this might be primarily for the benefit of the profession's standing, it also speaks of a responsible attitude to the public with a concern not to delude.

This concern carries over into the prohibition of specific therapeutic claims and offers in advertisements. On the one hand, it is fairer to the prospective patients, but, on the other, it is also good professional sense, safeguarding the membership from scientific and legal criticism. In Britain it perhaps makes legal sense not to mention diseases treated, as there are several which the law forbids non-medical practitioners to claim to treat. These include various venereal diseases, cancer and tuberculosis among others. The position which the naturopaths take philosophically, by not offering 'cure', takes on another dimension in this context. Many patients with cancers have sought out naturopathic help: their practitioners carefully state that they may only help improve the patient's general health, and make no claims to cure cancer.

The latter example perhaps demonstrates the way a group develops concepts of therapeutic responsibility as they arise within particular social circumstances. It is not possible for a group of practitioners to develop these ideas in a vacuum, nor for such concepts to be fixed in time. There are legal constraints on how and what one may practise in different settings: in Britain these are to do with the particular legal rules surrounding patients, doctors and practitioners. What the patient chooses to do may be challenged in the courts, particularly where someone refuses treatment that a doctor considers best for them. This is most obviously highlighted in the case of minors (who may be made wards of court and compelled to take medical treatment) and those adults thought to be incapable of making conscious and reasoned decisions. It is possible that on occasion relatives and friends feel that the very choice of a path as unorthodox as nature cure indicated mental instability on the patient's part. Where life apparently hangs in the balance with the terminally ill, practitioners may be strongly challenged as to whom they are responsible. However, these are not situations peculiar to naturopaths (see Kennedy, 1988).

Having found the formal rules on professional conduct so thin in the ISRN Bye-Laws I looked at other ethical codes, notably of the British Psychological Society (BPS) and the British Sociological Association (BSA). Before getting involved in an in-depth comparative study, serendipitously a newsletter from Consumers for Ethics in Research (CERES) came my way in which Ruth Wilkins had written a comparative review of just these guidelines. Her discussion opened with the question: 'If I was a research subject, with whom would I prefer to work?' She found the psychologists' guidelines apparently 'more rigorous but . . . shot through with morally questionable presumptions that need closer scrutiny' (Wilkins, 1991: 2). The latter were to do with the reliance at base on ' "strict controls and the disinterested approval of independent advisers" ', commenting 'What constitutes "independence" is anybody's guess, especially given our deference to science and medicine' (Wilkins, 1991: 2). She preferred the honesty of the sociologists' approach which jettisoned

> the concept of 'independent advice' favoured by the psychologists in favour of individual responsibility based on a set of ethical principles which, they note, should be departed from as a result of 'deliberation not ignorance'. That is, they trust no-one but themselves.
>
> (Wilkins, 1991: 2)

In conclusion Wilkins decided she preferred the latter's 'emphasis on values and individual responsibility' but felt that this placed 'high burdens on the researcher and [ran] significant risks of abuse and lack of accountability' (1991: 3).

I found a parallel here with my work in naturopathic practice, where the way is not signposted and sometimes the responsibilities in practice feel awesome. I hope that when I 'leave alone' it is by 'deliberation and not ignorance', but how sure can I be that I shall know when I am ignorant? I am always learning. We can say to ourselves as practitioners, in the way that Wilkins did above: 'If I was a patient, with whom would I prefer to work?' I am helped to answer that question for myself through a sequence of statements by Bertram T. Fraser, an Edinburgh-trained naturopath, that could be addressed to every patient:

> Nothing I ask you to do, or do for you, will do you any harm;
> Nothing I ask you to do, or do for you, will you not find pleasurable, if not at first, eventually;

Nothing I ask you to do, or do for you, am I not already doing myself, or am prepared to have done to me.

(Fraser, *c.*1948/9, quoted by H. Harrison, 1991)

These simple sentences contain the essence of responsible naturopathic practice, where the practitioners themselves continue to work at their own 'cure', applying 'nature care' in their own lives. Not many forms of modern health care can promise such a standard of both personal experience and no harm. (Shiatsu practice, Alexander, Tai Ch'i and Yoga teachers are analogous examples.)

However, Fraser's statement leaves us apparently entirely at the mercy of the individual practitioner's integrity, and mentions nothing of the way that an accountable standard of practitioner behaviour is evolved by a group. We still say Fraser's words to our patients, although the actual instructions we give today may well have altered slightly in the light of more recent research into nutrition and fasting, for example. Also, the type of medication available to patients through their general practitioners constantly changes and it is imperative that naturopaths keep up to date with their knowledge of drug side-effects, interactions and the effects of withdrawal (gradual or sudden), so that safe and responsible clinical decisions may be made. Keeping informed is part of one's therapeutic responsibility, and here the membership of a professional body, attendance at conferences and training sessions, as well as more informal contact with colleagues is essential.

Some comments on a recent study of osteopathic competence are equally relevant to the naturopathic profession:

The thing to realize is that the criteria [of minimum levels of competence] do not exist in some filing cabinet or book: the . . . [naturopathic] profession itself must decide on them and construct them.

(Sketchley, 1992)

Constructing and deciding upon criteria to do with therapeutic responsibility can be seen as an ever ongoing process, a discourse, with many participants. In some ways, as we have seen from this brief review of written codes, ultimately the ethical issues around our therapeutic responsibility can only be resolved at the 'coal face' in the particular patient–practitioner relationship. It is to the relationship aspect of the 'healing bond' that we now turn.

A relationship

We have reiterated the motto 'only nature heals', but we cannot ignore the human nature of the healing bond. The emotional bond between patient and practitioner probably cannot be codified. We move into a discussion that recognizes the ragged edges of practice. I have used Peter Fenton's (1987) paper 'Therapeutic Relationship – A Naturopathic Viewpoint' for a number of points in this section. To organize the material I raise issues about the relationship as they would arise perhaps in the first consultation with a patient.

My first contact with the patient may be by telephone or letter. Very often the process of re-definition mentioned above starts here, when we explain that we offer no cure, but try to understand the person's presenting complaints or concerns from primary causes. Many practitioners send nature cure literature to the patient with the booking confirmation, so that a better understanding of the approach can commence before the first meeting. Occasionally people will cancel at this point, deciding that nature cure is not what they want. Some practitioners ask the patient to send back a potted life and health history so as to gain an insight as to the reason for the consultation, and, importantly, a view of the way the patient sees their life.

The first consultation starts usually with the practitioner asking for information such as name, address, date of birth, occupation. Even at this stage the way in which we ask questions affects the nature of the relationship. Not everyone likes to give their date of birth and this has to be respected. Asking the patient what title they use is preferable to the presumptuous 'Is it Miss or Mrs?' still so commonly asked of a woman. The way we ask questions throughout the history-taking can avoid sexism, hetero-sexism and racism. For example, it may indeed be relevant to inquire in some detail into the arrangements for eating and cooking if we hope to effect changes along nature cure lines. Asking 'Do you live alone/cater for yourself?' is preferable to the questions 'Are you married/ does your wife cook for you?' which assume hetero-sexism and gender divisions of domestic labour. The careful use of wording in questions makes a lot of difference to the way in which patients feel accepted as whole people.[6] It is from this feeling of being accepted and cared about that the therapeutic relationship can start. There must be respect for the person in the context of their culture, their occupation, their social and family life. This is realistic if we are to help them through the inevitable traumas of change-making that we may deem clinically necessary for them to get some movement back towards 'high-level health'. In contrast, some patients come to a first consultation already feeling that they know me, thanks to an enthusiastic friend or relation of theirs who has told them all about their own experience.

After the initial questions the patient is encouraged to describe the main reasons that have brought them to us at this particular time. It is our responsibility to listen very carefully, not just for the bare bones of clinical data, but also to aspects of the story that tell us what the situation means for this particular patient. We can also 'listen . . . for what the patient doesn't say either by inference or demonstrable gestures' (Fenton, 1992). When we ask further questions to enable us to put the current picture in the context of the patient's lifestyle and history, we try to focus on the healing episodes of their lives rather than the disease crises. Again, we are committed to reframing the view that the person has of themselves, by encouraging them to start loving, respecting and trusting their bodies. So, for example, when a heavy smoker says apologetically that they frequently have a productive cough, we say 'Good! the lungs are still busy trying to throw out the muck!' We may add that we are more concerned about those people who come along saying triumphantly that they never have a day's illness, when it is clear from the tally of lifestyle debts they have accumulated that the body's vital capacity was diminished long ago and would not dare to risk even a mild healing crisis such as a head cold. But here we also have a responsibility to observe the non-verbal communication and to judge the sensitivity of the patient. Not everyone will feel comfortable with the comments above and those people's needs also have to be respected.

When we move on to the physical examination we must accept what the patient feels comfortable with in terms of undress. Obviously it is difficult, for example, to examine the spine when it is completely covered up, but for those patients who are genuinely uncomfortable undressing in front of strangers, clothing may often be strategically moved to expose a few vertebrae at a time. There is a balance to be struck between therapeutic responsibility in terms of respecting the patient's needs for dignity, and their needs for adequate diagnosis and treatment. It is not good clinical practice, for example, to test the plantar responses[7] through the socks, stockings or tights! There are also the situations where the patient has little regard for the comfort of the practitioner, and diplomatic assertiveness is a skill worth cultivating.

The physical examination and any physical treatment deemed appropriate are potentially areas for great vulnerability for the patient and the practitioner. For the patient, it may be the only time that they are touched, except by their sexual partner/s or very close friends. For the practitioner, the modern world of increasing litigation should have brought an awareness of the need for clarity. For both the patient's and the practitioner's sake it is important that the naturopath explains what examinations will be carried out and why, in simple language that the patient can understand. If there are examinations that might be found personal or intrusive, such as a rectal or vaginal examination, or, say, the palpation of the groin, the purpose of these examinations should be clearly explained and the patient asked whether they mind these being carried out. Often in my own practice I will ask patients if they would feel more comfortable having a rectal or vaginal examination carried out by their general practitioner or practice nurse. If they would prefer this, I then write to the National Health surgery explaining why I think such an examination would be helpful, and usually this works out well. It is one way of coping with the dilemma that making a differential diagnosis poses in some cases. It could be a serious omission on my part were I not to make sure that, for example, the prostate gland was normal and not enlarged. It would be relinquishing therapeutic responsibility.

Apart from these very private examinations, the whole issue of the way I touch the patient is relevant to any discussion of therapeutic responsibility. I must recognize that touching someone at all is a special form of communication, and often I will make such contact with a patient early on with a handshake as they enter my practice. This is part of our first communication and can establish a mood or offer reassurance. Later, during the case-history-taking I ask about aspects of general health such as the quality of circulation, at which point I usually want to look at the hands and nails so we make physical contact again. In this way there is a preparation for the full physical examination. If I or the patient feels uncomfortable about the examination I must respect this and either delay any examination for another meeting, or refer elsewhere if this is appropriate. During the examination I usually comment on positive signs of health as part of the process of encouraging the patient to trust the healing power of their body.

At the summing up of the findings from this first meeting, Fenton writes of prognoses:

> we are trying to define the indefinable – and there are so many variables – but in Nature Cure, in so far as we give prognoses, we give the *optimum* prognosis consistent with the patient's age, vital capacity and degree of degeneration and reason for living.
>
> (1987: 14; emphasis in original)

The naturopath sees a responsibility to encourage healing in the patient, and stressing the optimum prognosis is one way of engendering hope in the patient, which in itself has a life-enhancing effect. Fenton contrasts this with the 'more dismal' prognosis in medicine, which he says is 'partly because of the suppressive methods used and partly because there was no adjustment in the patient's lifestyle' (1987: 14).

Another aspect of hope-giving to the patient is through non-verbal communication. I have already mentioned the careful way in which a relationship through touch must be established, and touching in a caring and confident manner communicates acceptance and encouragement to the patient. Fenton also talks about a more subtle non-verbal communication that comes from our own ideation.

He describes how, when he examined a woman who had been somewhat mutilated by a mastectomy, she had picked up his immediate thoughts though he had not spoken:

> How do we prevent this non-verbal communication in a negative sense – it must occur positively. Only by treating the patient on his/her own merits without colouring from the past (especially failures). An openness without final conclusions – visualize the patient as you wish them to be – but the mind is always weighing, measuring, comparing, projecting and forecasting.
>
> (Fenton, 1987: 17)

A combination of outward affirmation of the patient is required alongside an inward reflection on one's practice. Responsible practitionership implies this commitment to an ongoing reflection upon oneself and thereby one's relationships with all patients. Our knowledge-base must also include an honest appraisal of our limitations as practitioners, both as individual people with our own emotional histories, and as naturopaths, when we are working close to the boundaries of our expertise. Sometimes it may be responsible to refer our patient on to another sort of practitioner, or to have the supervision of a more experienced naturopath.

In the ISRN postgraduate course recently we have been exploring our images of the patient–practitioner relationship: there are many (Power, 1991). The following emerged in group discussion at an ISRN seminar in Malvern in 1992:

Practitioner's role	Patient's role
healer	someone in need
intellectual/reasoning	'student'
authority figure	obedient servant
saviour	victim to be saved
mother/father	child
providing knowledge	student/ally
confidante	confessor
example setter	student/pupil/mirror
encourager	struggler
loving carer	receiver
servant (in NHS)	master/litigator

No doubt there are more possibilities. We have agreed in our conference and teaching discussions with students and practitioners that 'we don all these hats according to the circumstances' (Fenton, 1987: 15).

I have decided to use the last section of this chapter for a series of examples from practice, to give flesh to the somewhat idealistic bones I have attempted to sketch out in the two sections above. I think that both aspects of the 'healing bond', the contract and the relationship, come through these.

RESPONSIBILITY IN PRACTICE

Let us start with the most formal aspects of responsibility: say a situation that any practitioner would dread where their professional membership is threatened because of complaints from patients. How is the profession 'policed'? I gleaned a couple of examples from the past. These involved complaints about male practitioners' attire during treatment. One case Fenton (1992) cites was of working in orange robes, the other in bathing trunks. Some female patients in particular found the lack of a formal clinic coat threatening. The first approach by the Society has tended to be informal, contacting the practitioner concerned to discuss matters in confidence. Fenton (1992) writes:

> in both cases whilst recognizing the need for individual expression the practitioner is imposing his personality/beliefs/lifestyle . . . to an unjustified and unwarranted extent.

However, these examples merely skirt (trouser?) a far more serious issue: that of sexual harassment or 'unethical intimacy' (Garrett and Thomas-Peter, 1992) in the practitioner–patient encounter. Most commonly this would be a male practitioner harassing a female patient. This has not been a subject openly raised in training nor at annual conferences. It is well known but not publicly acknowledged. A woman colleague commented:

> the odd weirdo practising in idiosyncratic garb doesn't really do justice . . . [to the issue]. [Sexual harassment] . . . definitely exists and it is something the profession ought to acknowledge, especially as in the alternative medicine setting there is too much room for misinterpretation of a situation on the one hand (why the complete body exam for a headache, where this is clinically justified) and dubious behaviour on the other (palpating *every* woman's breasts, in case the back pain is associated with breast malignancies. Justifiable sometimes, but not as a rule). The guidelines are loose, the practitioner most of the time works by her/himself.

(de Quiros, 1992)

What sanctions could be applied if the practitioner did not comply with their professional organization's recommendations? The ultimate sanction would be the removal of membership. What this would mean in terms of the effect on practice in Britain is probably not very significant in a situation where there are many naturopathic organizations and the public are not well-informed about these. In a monopoly situation, like the British Medical Association, such a sanction would carry much more weight, and mean that the practitioner would not get insured and so on. However, in the small and diverse naturopathic field, the membership of a group can be significant both for mutual referrals and for the ongoing support that professionals give each other, so the threat of the loss of these could be sufficient.

There has been a system of reviewing the practices of new members of the ISRN, both to ensure that the basic rules are being kept, and, more positively, to offer support and help. This usually involves visits to one's practice on a fairly informal basis. During my first year in membership, I received a visit from a senior naturopath who sat in on several of my sessions with patients who had given permission for the intrusion. One woman patient enjoyed receiving some treatment from both of us at once, as we each massaged one of her legs! I believe that there have been a few practitioners who have been asked not to renew their membership when they have continued to use 'adjuncts' despite discussion. Some individuals have removed themselves from membership because they themselves felt they could not continue in all conscience under the stringent codes quoted above. Apart from such 'inspections' there is an expectation within the Society that one will attend conferences and seminars at fairly regular intervals.

Despite the basic commitment to avoid the use of supplementation, most naturopaths accept that there are rare occasions when it can positively affect the healing process. We would explain to the patient that this is a temporary phase and no part of cure or long-term 'nature care'. There are particular situations where it would be clinically irresponsible to remove the patient's existing props without long-term improvements in feeding, rest, breathing, exercise and so on. Pregnancy is a good example where it could be positively dangerous to mother and baby's health to make big dietetic changes in mid-term. It is quite different when working with a patient who has been living a nature cure lifestyle for a number of years prior to pregnancy. I am not saying that no naturopathic advice or help may be given to women who first consult in pregnancy, but am stressing that this needs to be given with cautious reference to the full health history, family history, and so on.

Generally, in a rather compromised situation, where there has been much reliance on conventional medication, supplementation and/or homoeopathic or herbal preparations for some years, one treads with caution in an unknown and unpredictable field. There is no question that antibiotic therapy can sometimes be genuinely life-saving, and therefore 'buy time' for the patient. This was the case with a young man who presented for first consultation with a serious case I diagnosed as pneumonia. I told him to go to hospital immediately. This action was against his initial wishes as he had valiantly 'fasted' on fruit alone for more than two months, without supervision, and came wanting immediate naturopathic care. In the non-residential clinic setting I knew I could not provide the extensive care that he needed, but continued to build a relationship with him in the hospital.

Very often patients come after they have undergone a number of orthodox interventions which we would see as having seriously suppressed their vitality. This is particularly so in the conventional treatment of cancers. Radiotherapy is a case in point. Where tissue has been irradiated it is highly probable that one is dealing with not only areas of dead tissue, but surrounding cells and structures that may be alive but are functioning abnormally as a result of radiation. One patient with AIDS who had suffered from Kaposi's sarcoma on the legs had had the growths 'killed' by radiation, but was still suffering from the after-effects with massive swelling around the lower legs, feet and ankles. I had to make a decision about what, if any, intervention was safe. Local massage would be contraindicated, and even cold water paddling might be too active an intervention and stir up a crisis situation that this particular patient might not be able to handle. We discussed the safest route to healing, as I shared my cautious but positive thinking, and we mutually decided that nutritional improvements might come first, along with a commitment to seek more rest and to attempt to cut down on life-depleting habits such as smoking. To help the latter I taught some simple relaxation techniques, which this particular patient took further by seeking out a course in auto-suggestion. There were crises and fortunately I was able to home visit on a couple of occasions, and to keep in contact by phone to some extent.

Responsibility as a naturopath has to extend beyond the clinic walls and this means being available by telephone at most times. This can be a daunting commitment when first qualified as one's own home life (e.g. bed, breakfast, baths and supper) are repeatedly interrupted. A balance has to be learned for one's own survival (and that of one's nearest and dearest) and the use of the answerphone is a great boon. Having a specific time available for telephone consultations is also very helpful. Here I should stress that such 'consultations' are strictly not available to patients who have never been seen. This is another aspect of responsible practice. It is genuinely dangerous to diagnose over the telephone, and even where I know a patient well I will recommend a second opinion from a casualty department or a general practitioner in certain circumstances, if neither myself nor a colleague can be at hand for consultation or a home visit.

Inevitably, conflicting situations may arise for the patient who has consulted both a naturopath and a doctor, who may fundamentally disagree on diagnosis and also on treatment. 'Straight' naturopaths see themselves as an alternative both to medicine and to most of what has been called 'complementary' medicine. Where I have suggested a patient attend the hospital or visit a general practitioner for an opinion or a further investigation (e.g. X-rays or blood tests) I make it clear that the patient does not have to accept the conventional treatment that may be offered, and that usually there is time for us to discuss the implications of that treatment and those of the naturopathic approach. It may be considered that in taking this line I am making the patient unduly dependent on myself and upon a minority view of health and illness. The latter is true but I challenge the criticism. Carol Smith (1983), a naturopath who made a special study of naturopathic gynaecology, stressed that women are already under so much pressure within the orthodox system to comply without asking questions about the dangers of treatment that it was essential that we discuss in simple terms a range of possibilities, and stress the usual safety of the naturopathic approach. These situations underline our need to keep up-to-date at a basic level with current medical practice as well. An interesting parallel has recently been raised by an osteopath discussing malpractice litigation (albeit in rather a defensive tone):

> osteopaths today, to protect themselves in the eyes of the law, should give each new patient a reasonable account of their condition, the osteopathic treatment they are going to receive, its probable length, discomforts, likelihood of success and alternative treatments available. Otherwise patients may turn round at a later stage and say 'I would not have undertaken this treatment had I known it was going to be so painful/last so long/would not be 100% successful or could have been replaced by drug treatment.' On the other hand there is the fascinating possibility that patients in future will be in a position to sue orthopaedic surgeons who carry out spinal surgery without informing their patients beforehand of the possible benefit of non-invasive osteopathic treatment!
>
> (Norfolk, 1992: 3)

The mind genuinely boggles at the thought of queues of litigants complaining about the effects of, say, life-long steroid treatment for eczema, holding that the general practitioner should have discussed with them the various possibilities of, say, naturopathy, or homoeopathy or herbalism. Many other startling scenarios can be envisioned should such a future ever come to be. Perhaps I am pessimistic, or realistic, when I suspect that as part of a responsible attitude to practice we will still do the major part of the explanation and education work with patients. One reality for most general practitioners in the British National Health Service is just not having enough time – obviously there are notable exceptions – and maybe we see many patients whom the system has failed.

I cannot see that the future holds out a significant change in power relationships between naturopaths and doctors for all the talk of cooperation and complementarity. The medical profession is straightforwardly more powerful on almost every dimension that one may care to measure, and any legal definition of what a doctor should tell the patients is likely to be formulated in collusion between doctors and lawyers, not naturopaths and lawyers.

Nevertheless, there are some advantages to being in a marginal position and this leads me to a broader series of points about therapeutic responsibility. I have highlighted the personal commitment by the naturopath to the care of their own health, and have illustrated some of their concerns for the patient. Growing out of these personal and clinical concerns flows a critique of a status quo that maintains a situation where huge numbers of people in the world have no access to the most basic nutrition, and a large number in the West are made sick by over-nutrition and 'empty' nutrition or 'junk food'. At root this is to do with a long history of both human and environmental exploitation globally. Among the naturopaths it is usual to find the concept of responsibility stretching far out beyond the walls of the practice into concerns for society, for the political world and for the earth itself. Obviously the specific nature of these concerns held by individual naturopaths varies enormously. Some are overtly active in various organizations while others support and aid many concerns (e.g. Greenpeace, the Soil Association, the Vegetarian Society, Friends of the Earth, the Anti-Apartheid Movement, the Campaign for Nuclear Disarmament, the Peace Pledge Union and so on). There is evidence of a long tradition of involvement with outgoing concerns of a very varied nature, as Julia Twigg (1982) reported in her study of the social history of vegetarianism. Famous nature cure supporters and enthusiasts in Britain have included Bernard Shaw and A.S. Neill (of Summerhill, the 'free school', fame).

However, for the individual patient–practitioner relationship it is advisable that one's political involvements are in the main kept private from the immediate clinical setting, so naturopathy proves accessible to all, another aspect of responsibility. As part of their healing process many patients become interested in wider issues, such as agribusiness when searching for additive-free, non-processed foods at the local supermarket. Increasingly, as 'green' issues have come to be placed on a world agenda, patients have come actively seeking naturopathy as a 'green' approach to health care. I find it very satisfying to feel that my work can touch on such a breadth of concerns. We sometimes ask if the practitioner acts as catalyst in the healing situation: I think it works both ways, and working with people in a nature cure practice is a continually encouraging and surprising experience for me as practitioner as well.

CONCLUSION

We have looked at the idea of a 'healing bond' in nature cure practice, both as a contract and as a human relationship, and I have shared some examples. I hope I have successfully conveyed my experience both as an individual practising in an English context, and as a member of the Incorporated Society of Registered Naturopaths. Many of the points I have touched on are common to all who work in health care professions. Where I feel nature cure is distinctive is in the 'intelligent leaving alone', the non-doing, and the refusal to recognize any source of 'cure' other than 'nature'. This 'letting be' is maybe more prevalent in the psychotherapies or spiritual guidance. It is a challenging aspect of naturopathic practice when a patient comes demanding specific treatments. As practitioners we have to accept that we may 'lose' patients to other complementary therapists who are prepared to give 'cures' in response to demand. I would not feel accountable to myself if I did not attempt some 'reframing' of the concepts of health and illness with most patients. I would be untrue to the saying: 'only nature heals'.

NOTES

The author would like to acknowledge the help of Áine Collins and Peter Fenton for critical advice with this chapter.

1 Fenton (1992) comments: 'the earlier naturopaths distanced themselves maximally from medicine and remedies and symbolism and the "mixers" compromise this situation philosophically and therapeutically.'

2 Fenton (1992) comments: 'If the patient is clinically alive then a healing capacitance is present reflected in the flow of blood and the beating of the heart etc.' What constitutes 'clinically alive' is also subject to ongoing debate, however, as Kennedy (1988) indicates in his discussions regarding, for example, switching off life-support machines.

3 Ian Kennedy (1988: 315–26), writing from a legal point of view, has stated that the 'relationship between doctor and patient is regulated by agreement between the two parties' in Continental Europe and in the United States, but pointed out that this is not the case in England. There he held that there is no contract between doctor and patient because of the availability of medical care through the National Health Service. He said that the idea of a contract with its implication that medicine is a commodity is 'a notion specifically rejected in England'. Obviously to date this has not been the case for the majority of naturopaths in England, so like the practitioner–patient relationship in the rest of Europe and the United States, we may talk of contracts.

4 Fenton (1992) comments: 'A distinction here is being made (to perhaps preempt medical or other criticisms of vitalist approaches) between intelligent leaving alone and criminal negligence, that is to say, a practitioner would not leave to nature's beneficence e.g. status epilepticus, status asthmaticus, fracture of the middle meningeal artery, serious comminuted fractures or vital obstruction, etc.'

5   This attitude to hypnotism may perhaps be traced to the distrust of 'mesmerism'
    (hypnotism as practised by Mesmer) by some in the Victorian movements of
    physical puritanism (a significant historical background to straight nature cure).
    Harrison wrote of the rejection of mesmerism:

> Mesmerism carried sexual overtones because of the fear of one person
> dominating another, especially if the mesmerist was a man and the subject a
> young woman.

(J. Harrison, 1987: 211)

Fenton (1992) raises another issue, with which I disagree:

> Hypnotism involves a form of evolutionary regression . . . whereas nature cure
> involves self-discipline, self-knowledge and expansion of consciousness.

I argue that 'self-knowledge' for some may only be accessed at first through this
sort of regression. The debate goes on!

6   Fenton (1992) adds: 'one must avoid anything initially which is perceived as
    inquisitive until the patient's confidence is gained – a gentle respect whilst
    trying to elicit sufficient facts to come to a differential diagnosis – we cannot
    gain all the information necessary at a first appointment. The patient must feel
    "I'm safe here – this is a framework/relationship in which I can get better".
    Often all a patient wants to know is that recovery *is* possible, especially regard-
    ing terminal or negative processes.'

7   The plantar response is that produced by scratching the undersurface of the foot up
    the long outside edge and then along towards the big toe. The direction of the
    involuntary reflex movement of the big toe in adults should normally be downwards,
    into flexion. If it moves upwards, it can be an important neurological sign.

REFERENCES

Crawford, R. (1980) 'Healthism and the Medicalization of Everyday Life', *International Journal of Health Services*, 10(3): 365–88.

de Quiros, S. (1992) Personal communication from a professional colleague, August.

Fenton, P. (1987) 'Therapeutic Relationship – A Naturopathic Viewpoint', paper
given at a seminar of the Incorporated Society of Registered Naturopaths,
Malvern Nature Cure Centre, Great Malvern, November.

Fenton, P. (1992) Personal communication commenting on an early draft of this
chapter.

Garrett, T. and Thomas-Peter, B. (1992) 'Sexual Harassment', *The Psychologist*,
July: 319–21.

Harrison, H. (1991) Personal communication from the president of the ISRN.

Harrison, J. (1987) 'Early Victorian Radicals and the Medical Fringe', in W.
Bynum and R. Porter (eds), *Medical Fringe and Medical Orthodoxy*, London:
Croom Helm.

Kennedy, I. (1988) *Treat Me Right: Essays in Medical Law and Ethics*, Oxford:
Clarendon.

Larkin, G. (1983) 'Orthodox Medicine and Professional Control', paper given to
the Medical Sociology Group (of the British Sociological Association), annual
conference, University of York, September.

Muirhead, M. (1992) 'Nature Cure Philosophy', unpublished lecture given to the Postgraduate Training Course in Naturopathy, seminar III, of the Incorporated Society of Registered Naturopaths and the James C. Thomson Memorial Trust, Malvern Nature Cure Centre, Great Malvern, 28 February–2 March.

Norfolk, D. (1992) 'Malpractice Litigation, Part 3', *OAGB (Osteopathic Association of Great Britain) Newsletter*, June, 4(6): 3.

Power, R. (1984) 'A Natural Profession? – Issues in the Professionalization of British Nature Cure, 1930 to 1950', unpublished MSc dissertation, Polytechnic of the South Bank, London.

Power, R. (1989) *Specialists of the Natural, 1930–1950*, Health and Social Services Research Unit, Research Papers, no. 3, London: Polytechnic of the South Bank.

Power, R. (1991) 'Psychology 1', an unpublished lecture given to the ISRN postgraduate course, Great Malvern, November.

Rakusen, J. (1989) 'Alternative and Complementary Approaches to Health and Healing', in A. Phillips and J. Rakusen (eds), *The New Our Bodies, Ourselves* (British edition), Harmondsworth: Penguin.

Roth, J. and Hanson, R. (1976) *Health Purifiers and Their Enemies*, London: Croom Helm.

Sketchley, J. (1992) Letter accompanying a draft of *Competences Required for Osteopathic Practice*, Summer.

Smith, C. (1983) Lecture series in 'Naturopathic Gynaecology' given to the fourth-year students at the British College of Naturopathy and Osteopathy, London.

Thomson, C.L. (1966) *Living with Nature Cure*, Edinburgh: Kingston Publications.

Thomson, J. (n.d.) *The Belfast Lecture: The Way to High Level Health*, Edinburgh: Kingston Publications.

Twigg, J. (1982) 'The Vegetarian Movement in England 1847–1981, with Particular Reference to Its Ideology', unpublished PhD thesis, London School of Economics, University of London.

Wilkins, R. (1991) 'Ethics in Social Research: A Guide to the Guidelines', *CERES (Consumers for Ethics in Research) News*, Autumn/Winter, 8: 2–3.

10 Doctor and patient in family planning and psychosexual therapy

Gillian Vanhegan

My work in gynaecology, family planning and specialist psychosexual clinics creates an involvement between doctor and patient which is relatively unusual in orthodox medicine. In the latter two clinic settings the patients are rarely 'ill' in the conventional sense. Often they come with a particular choice that they have made or wish to make – to decide whether or not to have an abortion, to use contraception, to be able to have intercourse. They may wish to confine the doctor whom they see to a narrow technical role of someone who will provide them with an appropriate service. This may be all that they require, in which case the doctor can confine herself to the physical doctor role. Other cases need treatment on a deeper psychotherapeutic level and the doctor must be alert to her change of role for these patients.

Many physical problems in gynaecology, such as particularly heavy menstrual periods, are dealt with in a conventional way. The patient is examined for signs of anaemia and a pelvic examination is carried out to determine the normality of the uterus or the presence of fibroids. The necessary haematological investigations and pelvic scans are instigated. The results are collated and the doctor decides upon the best line of treatment, either medical or surgical.

The doctor is being a conventional gynaecologist, but should at no time forget the patient's feelings, especially with regard to hysterectomy and how the patient views the loss of her uterus. Some patients react with relief to the end of the anxieties related to the risk of pregnancy. Others will be distressed at the loss of what they view as their femininity.

These patients have presented a problem to the doctor and accept the treatment which is offered. In the same way, the majority of patients attending family planning clinics only seek professional help in controlling their fertility. Methods of contraceptions are discussed with them, and they are given whatever is suitable for their needs. They have used the doctor as a professional and accepted her advice.

However, a number of patients attending doctors have problems of dis-ease (discomfort) at a deeper level, and the doctor must be constantly aware of their distress. The patient can have difficulty in admitting to her problem or verbalizing it. Many doctors, and especially those trained by the Institute of Psychosexual Medicine, remain alert to the unspoken word and the feeling in the consulting room. The doctor has a dual role of providing a strictly physical medical diagnosis and treatment, and/or working with the patient's deeper problems. The course of the consultation is ultimately directed by the patient, who is not always ready to look at the emotional causation of dis-ease. The interpretation of the relationship between doctor and patient is part of the therapy.

The following cases illustrate how I use the constantly changing doctor–patient bond during the course of treatment. The patients' names, physical descriptions and occupations have been altered to protect their anonymity.

CONSULTATION IN THE CASE OF AN UNPLANNED PREGNANCY

The patient presenting to a gynaecologist with her unplanned pregnancy is in a vulnerable situation. She has her own feelings of guilt – 'It's all my fault' – or anger – 'My boyfriend shouldn't have let this happen'. Her anxiety is compounded by not knowing the views of the doctor she consults, or being unable to define her wishes for the outcome of the consultation.

The setting for her consultation is beyond her control. She could be seen in the middle of a busy hospital gynaecology clinic by a registrar, who has rushed from a traumatic and overrunning operating list with no time for midday sustenance. This is the worst possible scenario and damaging for both patient and doctor. In this consultation the doctor's own pressures can be experienced by the patient and she would feel under pressure to reach a rapid decision about her pregnancy. She would not have had the opportunity to consider all the options open to her: continuing with her pregnancy, keeping the child, adoption or abortion.

A preferable setting for this patient's consultation would be a clinic, where time is allowed for discussion and the expression of her feelings about the pregnancy. Then the patient would have a doctor who is open-minded and non judgemental, leaving her able to express the often contradictory feelings of not wanting to continue with the pregnancy, but also not agreeing with termination. Surely this is the opportunity for her to express her fantasies surrounding abortion.

The patient–doctor relationship has to be one of trust, so that the patient has confidence to verbalize what can often be painful feelings. She has to trust the doctor not to betray her when she exposes her deepest feelings.

The patient is investing the whole of her future in the outcome of this consultation and has to have confidence that the doctor will help her reach a decision on the right line of action. She is looking not for a 'cure', but for a solution to her present dilemma. The patient needs information about the medical aspects of pregnancy and abortion, but also needs to express her own feelings.

The first case-history describes a young woman as she decides on an abortion, and the use that she makes of me as her doctor.

Julie attended the Youth Advisory Clinic with her boyfriend Gary. It was a cold November day and they had on their motorbike leathers, which made them appear well-defended against the world. However, a different picture emerged as they sat in the consulting room awaiting the result of a pregnancy test. He sat close to her, holding her hand in a way which was both loving and protective. I felt the strong caring bond between them and already saw the forthcoming difficulties disrupting their comfortable togetherness. The nurse looked through the door to confirm that the pregnancy test result was positive. Julie and Gary had had a strong suspicion that it would be but now they had to face up to the actuality. There was a moment of silent thought.

They had always used condoms, so they were able to express anger at the unfairness of the situation. I allowed them to verbalize the other feeling of amazement that their love-making had produced a potential new life. Gary stayed in the room whilst Julie was examined, and I noted that this was an extension of his need to care for her. Some boyfriends remain in an aggressive or offensive way to cross-examine the doctor, not trusting their girlfriend to report honestly what had happened in the examination room. Even after the examination Gary and Julie remained amazed and rather in awe of what had happened to them.

I felt I should lead them gently along the path to reality. Julie was only just 18 and spoke enthusiastically about the A-levels she would sit in June and her hopes of university and a career in mathematics. Her mother was a widow and had worked hard to bring up Julie and her brother, giving them the best educational opportunities. Gary was 24, although he looked younger, and was already well established in an artistic career. He lived with Julie at her home, as her mother approved of the relationship.

The magic of the moment of the confirmation of the pregnancy floated away as they spoke and they put me firmly in a physical-medical rule, with questions about the expected delivery date and problems during pregnancy. I was aware that I was being put into this role, but felt that this was not because they were trying to escape the emotional dilemma of the circumstances, but rather that they required practical medical information. After the consultation Julie and Gary were referred to a trained counsellor working in the clinic to give them more time for discussion with a third party. Armed with all the necessary information they left to consider their situation over the next few days.

This interval for thought is necessary so that the patient can reach her own decision. No decision should be reached in the panic which ensues after a positive pregnancy test result. Decisions made at this stage can lead to regret at a later date (Conway *et al.*, 1989: 13). During this first consultation the role of the doctor had been two-fold. There is the physical-doctor role, needed to ascertain the fitness of the patient, the period of gestation and to furnish the patient with purely medical information on pregnancy, childbirth, abortion and any other relevant factors. Running concomitantly is the role of the carer, who is not judging the patient, but helping her to verbalize her innermost feelings about her condition. The doctor moves between the two roles in response to the patient's needs. A high proportion of patients do not have the support of partner or family during the interval allowed for the decision-making. It is hoped that the doctor–patient relationship is a strong enough bond and that the patient will feel able to telephone with any queries. In Julie's case she had a great deal of support during her time for reflection.

At the next consultation Julie and Gary attended together and I noted that Julie looked older and tired. I commented on Julie's appearance, which opened the door for Julie to talk at length about her internal deliberations of the past few days. Julie decided that mentally she would be unable to cope with the intersecting and divisive lines of tension which would be created by the birth of a child during the same month as her A-level examinations. There had been no external pressures brought to bear on her decision, but only open-minded discussions around the table, between Julie, Gary, Julie's mother and brother. I sensed the care and time which had been spent on reaching the decision, and the good relationship which remained between Julie and Gary.

In my experience many shallow relationships are wrecked on the rocks of the crisis created by an unplanned pregnancy. I was also aware that a high proportion of patients who experience post-abortion distress are in marriages or ongoing partnerships. The carer's role does not finish at the time of the operation, as the healing bond will be required in the months which follow.

I was alerted to my role of care and protection when Julie returned alone for her post-abortion follow-up visit. I was greatly relieved to hear that Gary was working to meet a deadline with some creative artwork, and chastised myself for a moment when I had suspected him of desertion. There was no pain in the consulting room, but a feeling of completeness. Julie expressed no regrets, only positive feelings about the future of academic plans and her relationship with Gary. I noted that I was speaking to a more mature Julie than previously, but still left the consulting room door open for Julie to contact me if ever there were moments of regret. So far there have been none.

CONTRACEPTION AND THE ABUSED PATIENT

A patient attending for contraceptive advice has her own pre-conceived ideas on the options available, and her behaviour during the consultation can alert the doctor to the patient's fantasies and fears about her own sexuality. This is often most vivid when discussing the diaphragm or cap. Comments such as 'I couldn't put anything inside myself', 'I'm far too small for that' or 'Will it get lost?' show the patient's fantasies about her anatomy or her lack of readiness for sex. Some patients try to put the entire onus for sex on to their partners by choosing condoms as their only form of contraception.

The next case shows how a woman who appears asking for contraception is in fact asking for something else. If the doctor confines herself to the apparent need, she misses the real one. Such cases often make carers prickly and resentful, and it is important to be aware of this as a clue to how the patient is testing the doctor out before allowing a more dependent relationship to develop.

Ella presented in a busy family planning clinic. She apparently wanted contraception, but had negative comments on every method which she was offered. The combined oestrogen and progesterone oral contraceptive had made her gain weight and become depressed; a change to a different brand had given her headaches. She had also tried the minipill, which had disrupted her menstrual cycle. Several years previously she had had an intra-uterine coil, which had been removed within a few months of insertion, as Ella had complained of severe pain and heavy periods. So she refused to consider another coil. The thought of being instructed on the use of a diaphragm made her comment that she could not face the mess of jellies and creams and forethought needed to use this method. Finally she rejected the offer of an injectable depot of progesterone on the grounds that she had heard of unpleasant side-effects.

I began to feel that I was in receipt of a good deal of dissatisfaction and put it back to the patient that perhaps she was dissatisfied with her sexual life. Ella had appeared aggressive and dismissive in the first part of the consultation but now she displayed extreme anxiety, with twitching facial muscles. She choked out her distress at being unable to gain any stability or satisfaction in her sexual life. Whilst I had been in the role of the physical family planning doctor I had felt increasing annoyance with this 'problem' patient, who had been making unrealistic demands for the perfect contraceptive. Now the doctor–patient relationship became one of care and concern for an obviously anxious and distressed patient.

Ella was in her thirties and lived alone with her two school-age children. She was separated from her husband. She had a 'boyfriend' of about her own age, but could not allow herself a very close relationship with him, although physical intercourse did take place. I sensed the patient's need to withhold herself emotionally during intercourse and inquired gently if this had always been the case. With pain and difficulty Ella explained that her grandmother had brought her up when she was young. At the age of 9 she had gone back to her mother, who had remarried and had had another small daughter. The accommodation necessitated that Ella share a bedroom with her stepsister. Every night her stepfather came to say prayers over his daughter's bed, then moved on to Ella's bed where he abused her by manual manipulation of her genitals.

I allowed Ella to express how she found adult sexual foreplay distasteful and how she did not allow herself any excitation with her present partner in the same way as she had suppressed any excitement as a child. By early adolescence Ella had developed anorexia and could fit into extremely tight jeans which she wore to bed. When her stepfather discovered this line of defence, he merely said 'Good girl'. I suggested that this remark had made Ella feel yet more guilty about being previously more available. Ella looked like a small child again as she agreed with wide, sad eyes.

At the end of the consultation I was able to view the long road which Ella had walked down during the preceding half an hour. The prickly and aggressive patient had made the doctor try to find her satisfactory contraception. Once the doctor realized that the dissatisfaction was Ella's own feelings about her sex life, the door was opened for Ella to recount the pain of her childhood experiences. Often the patient who makes herself an uncomfortable person to be with can end up being rejected by reception, nursing and medical staff in a busy clinic, when it is easier to deal with a polite and conforming patient who readily accepts medical advice.

Before her second visit Ella phoned me to check the date and time of the consultation. I felt annoyed at this unnecessary manoeuvre, but was able to use this in the interpretation of the doctor–patient relationship. The doctor was an older woman, who had taken on the role of a caring mother-figure; Ella had needed to check that the doctor still cared enough to want to continue to help her as her own mother had not. Ella told me that her mother slept in the next room, but had never come to her aid when Ella had tried to shout during the abuse. In fact she had made her daughter available to her next partner. When Ella was 13 her mother had divorced the quasi-religious stepfather and was now living with another man. Abuse by this new man began when Ella had a cough and her mother had given the man a menthol compound to rub on her chest.

The devastating second period of abuse led to a pregnancy, which ended in a painful and bloody miscarriage when Ella was 14. I helped Ella to express all her feelings of dirt and pain arising from the abuse, and of her rejection, which culminated in Ella's mother utterly denying the situation, even when confronted with the miscarriage. Her mother made Ella's position in the family even more untenable as she showered affection on the stepsister both privately and at any possible public occasion.

I continued to act as an accepting and understanding mother-figure allowing Ella to work through her feelings of guilt and rejection. I was also able to praise and admire Ella as I realized the success she had made of her life. She had left home at the earliest opportunity, supporting herself with various jobs, and then trained to be a nurse. She supported herself and her two children, holding down a nursing job which involved long hours on duty. Sadly her marriage had foundered, as sex had not been a success and her husband had used her confession of abuse as a weapon against her in any argument. The second child had been delivered by a male midwife, which had caused distress beyond belief to the husband. He was unable to cope and confused the stepfather and abuser of her childhood with the male midwife. He left home when the baby was a few weeks old, saying that he could not stay with a woman who could be such a slut as to allow a man to touch her like that.

Over the next few visits I felt Ella became more able to put her childhood behind her and come to terms with life as an adult. She even managed to deal with a visit from her mother and the abuser of her childhood, who had wanted to babysit for her children. She had firmly kept him away from her children and I admired the way she could now say a firm 'no' to this figure who had terrified her. As Ella matured I was able to slide back into a physical role and examine her, even being able to take a cervical smear. Normally in a family planning clinic if the patient in her thirties had never had a smear test a doctor would have felt the need to do this test as soon as possible. In Ella's case I felt I would have been attacking or abusing what to the patient was a damaged private part of her anatomy. I was only able to examine her when the trauma of the abuse was left behind and Ella became a mature woman seeking contraception.

In fact she started an oral contraceptive pill and reported no problem at her following visit. Six months later, to my delight, Ella was pleased to say that her husband was coming back from Canada for a holiday to see her and the children. On the telephone he had suggested that if all went well he would like them to return to Canada with him. I shared Ella's pleasure, and allowed myself a few moments of happiness that my daughter/patient had grown up so well.

CONTRACEPTION AND THE INJURED PATIENT

The most difficult injury to help a patient with is one inflicted by a fellow-doctor. We never know whether the other doctor has in fact said or done the dreadful things which have injured the patient, or whether the incident has been embellished by the patient's own fantasies or mis-constructions. We are torn between defending a fellow-professional and hating him or her for inflicting harm. We must be aware of these contra-dictions before we can help our injured patient.

The next case-history is about a patient traumatized by previous medical treatment, which had had devastating effects on her sexual relationships. In this encounter the doctor has to use a mixture of counselling and practical skills to help the patient to overcome her inhibition.

When Anthea attended the family planning clinic for a repeat prescrip-tion of the contraceptive pill, I noted that she had been taking the pill for more than a year and suggested that she should have a cervical smear test. Anthea, who was a pretty, auburn-haired teacher, had been sitting rather demurely on her seat. At the mention of the smear test she crossed her legs in agitation and put her hands firmly and protectively in her lap. Tears welled in her eyes as she said that she had never had full intercourse. Gentle questioning made Anthea able to admit that she had been able to maintain a façade of normality as she lived with a gentle boyfriend who hoped that it would all be all right in the end. I sensed Anthea's deep distress as she said that her first boyfriend had also been rather meek and gentle and had not forced her to do anything she felt unable to do. She had loved him, but when she felt that she could never let him have sex with her she had used her new job in London as an opportunity to finish their relationship. She was happy with her new boyfriend, but sexual activity took the form of arousing each other to orgasm, with no penetration.

I was aware that Anthea remained closed to my questioning; she main-tained that nothing had ever happened to make her anxious about having sexual intercourse. She appeared to have a normal family background and a happy upbringing. She announced in a matter-of-fact way that she was unable to have sex, as her muscles were tight and closed. I realized that a psychosomatic examination of the vagina would be necessary to reveal the patient's subconscious feelings. The resistance which Anthea showed towards her boyfriend emerged with the doctor, and I felt it necessary to say that I would be as gentle as possible.

When the examination commenced, Anthea's whole body was rigid and her thighs were pressed firmly together. She said that she was unable to trust anyone, certainly not her boyfriend or myself, so I decided to put Anthea in charge of the examination by allowing her to guide my gloved hand. One fingertip was inserted into the vagina and then Anthea allowed it to advance about 2 cm, up to my first knuckle. At this point she withdrew my finger sharply and said 'That was horrible, I can't bear anything in my vagina. It reminds me of when I was 9 and my mother took me to the hospital.' She became increasingly distressed as she sat up and drew her knees into her body, rocking and wailing: 'she never warned me about the dreadful things that would happen to me.'

As a young child Anthea had had recurrent attacks of cystitis. Her mother was a nurse and had been anxious about this. Investigations had been arranged at the local hospital and it was necessary for a catheter to be inserted into the child's bladder so that dye could be injected for X-ray studies of the urinary tract. No anaesthetic had been given and Anthea had a vivid memory of nurses holding her down by her arms and legs whilst a doctor inserted the catheter. She remembered her thighs being forced apart and the ensuing pain as she had fought long and hard against the assault on her private parts. As she relived this agonizing memory she poured sweat which ran down her face and in rivulets across her chest; her final moan was 'Do you know if they still do this to children today?'

The patient was exhausted by the agony of reliving the pain of this incident. I allowed her to rail against the medical and nursing staff involved. There would have been nothing to gain by attempting to defend this group of professionals by remarks such as 'They were only doing their job' or 'They were doing what they thought was best for you'. Instead I chose to say: 'Yes, this awful thing has been done to you, and you will only be able to let someone into you when you feel ready, but you should not let this group of nurses and doctors win by ruining your life.'

At the next visit Anthea was more cheerful and pleased that she had used internal sanitary protection for the first time. She had been on holiday in a hot country, so it was something she had wanted to do to improve the quality of her life. I paid homage to Anthea's strength in being able to do something which she had previously found totally abhorrent. This was a more mature Anthea and she was able to work with me on her fear. Over the years Anthea had needed the physical barrier of vaginismus to protect the 'private parts' which had been invaded in childhood. The memory of extreme pain overlay fantasy, in which Anthea confused her urethra (urinary tract from the bladder) with her vagina. She expressed her ideas of the pain which would result if her boyfriend attempted to put his penis into this confused urethra/vagina.

This patient had tested the doctor and the doctor had remained gentle and trustworthy, not attacking and a source of pain as previous doctors had been. I had sensed from the moment that an examination had been suggested that the patient was terrified and had to be treated with great gentleness. In this atmosphere of trust the child-like patient had been able to talk about her injuries and fantasies. During the examination I treated the previously attacked private parts with respect and acknowledged that the patient owned this part of her body. Previously Anthea had felt that the control of this area had been handed over to her mother and the doctors and nurses. The more mature Anthea took command of her own genitals to use them as she saw fit and not to defend them for evermore. A doctor who is put in this role by the patient must not force the speed of consultation or examination or she will be seen as yet another uncaring medical practitioner.

THE MALE PATIENT AND FEMALE DOCTOR

It is not always women who seek help at a family planning clinic. Some men realize that it can be a place to go for help with sexual problems. These men have chosen not to visit their general practitioner with this problem; their doctor might be a friend or social acquaintance, especially in a small rural community. In this case the patient would be too embarrassed to approach his doctor with what he perceives as a highly personal problem. Such a man is convinced that he has an unusual problem and will often ask the psychosexual specialist in the family planning clinic 'Do you see many people with my problem?' This patient has decided that he has a problem, he has investigated where he can find help, and has been sufficiently motivated to make and keep an appointment. A female patient in a family planning clinic has an acceptable calling card, such as a request for contraception or cervical smear, and she presents this before her problem is revealed. A man will feel more exposed, as all he has to present is his problem. He expects to be seen by a female doctor in this setting, whereas if he sees a male doctor he might sense competition and feel the need to boast.

It is hoped that the male patient attends the clinic voluntarily, rather than being brought or sent by his partner. Research carried out by members of the Institute of Psychosexual Medicine has shown that the man who is motivated to seek help with a problem of impotence has a far higher cure rate than the unmotivated man (Lincoln and Thexton, 1979).

The next case-history shows how a man presenting with impotence alerts the doctor to its psychological origins by his passivity with her. When she is able to convince him that a firmer approach to his family relationships may make him feel more potent, his physical impotence is relieved. Here the doctor's stance is very important – she shows her patient by example that it is possible to stand up for yourself and make your mark. (The *double entendres* which crop up when we use metaphors about self-assertion are proof in themselves of the close links between physical and emotional potency.)

Peter was in his early forties, he was good looking and well dressed, but had an aura of sadness with drooping shoulders as he told me that he had been unable to make love to his wife for the last two years. He could not get an erection when he needed one, although he sometimes woke with one which disappeared as soon as he was conscious of it. He decided that he must have a physical problem, and I felt pushed into the role of being a conventional history-taking doctor. In fact Peter gave a normal medical history, with no serious operations, diseases or infections. Blood and urine analyses confirmed that he was fit. He seemed thankful to be examined and the genital examination revealed normal genitalia, which lay in an unresponsive way. I was used to male patients showing discomfort at examination or asking questions which show anxiety about the appearance of their genitalia. Sometimes the consultation and examination can be stimulating for the man and he has an erection, but Peter's passivity bordered on disinterest, and when I commented on this he admitted that he was disappointed that no physical cause for his impotence had been found.

When he was dressed again the consultation moved along the line of how easy it would be to take tablets to cure his problem and I realized how anxious he was about looking for psychological reasons. The sheer passivity which Peter had shown during examination made me comment that he wanted things done to him, such as being given tablets, but psychosexual therapy would require his participation. I noted my own frustration at a lack of feedback from this man and how I was becoming more demanding of the patient; and I put it to him that this must be the parallel situation to that between him and his wife. The patient revealed how he had no place in his own home. His wife led a busy life at her work all day and at her tennis club every night. His two teenage children never spoke to him and were either out with their friends or behind their firmly slammed bedroom doors. Whenever he attempted to criticize the teenagers' behaviour his wife took their side.

Peter had spent many years building his own company in a highly competitive area, so there had been times when he was away on business trips or just working late. During this time the family had developed a way of life which excluded him. I felt my frustration with this patient change to sympathy. I could see that his wife's rejection of him had led to his impotence. He would have to regain his position within the family and his standing with his wife to regain his potency.

Whilst I was explaining this to the patient, I was aware that I thumped the desk as I tried to instil determination into this passive man. The atmosphere lightened as I pointed out that Peter would be better when he could thump the desk and stand up for himself, both literally and physically, that is, with an erection. This had been the first time that Peter's anxieties had been acknowledged openly. His wife's frustration had made communication about Peter's worries impossible. Once the patient had been able to discuss his family problems with the doctor, he lost some of his sense of hopelessness and felt freed to talk to his wife again.

This case also illustrates how many patients, especially men, seek out a doctor with the expectation of physical treatment, but are able to use psychosomatic treatment. Peter was disappointed that his impotence did not have a physical explanation. He wanted to hand responsibility for his treatment to the doctor but there was no physical cause, so he had to participate in his treatment. The success or otherwise of a case is determined by the patient's ability to understand the interpretations of the healer–patient relationship, and to put what is learned from this into his sexual relationship. In other words, success lies in the hands of the patient more than the healer.

The next consultation saw a more confident Peter, who was proud of his achievements. He had been able to communicate with his wife, by making the effort to return home early enough to play tennis with her. He had harboured fantasies about her and other men at the tennis club, but when he had gone there with her he had been delighted by the way he was received and rather proud of his wife's good looks and behaviour. They had returned home and made love for the first time in two years. He had spoken to his wife about a new approach to the children's problems. At this point he even made a play of banging the desk to amuse me and emphasize his improvement.

During the consultation the doctor–patient relationship had changed to a meeting of equals, even of camaraderie, rather than the frustrated doctor and apathetic patient of the first meeting. The female doctor had been able to show the patient how his wife felt by studying the changing doctor–patient relationship. The man's improvement had been due to his motivation in seeking out a clinic suited to his problem; and in the way that he was able to understand and use the interpretations made during the consultation.

ADVISING YOUNG PATIENTS

The doctor working in a clinic which offers youth counselling and contraception must be aware of the different skills required when helping this age group. They are at an early stage in their sexual life and may often lack the basic knowledge and emotional stability to manage it. This ignorance and lack of confidence can often be hidden behind a façade of aggression, impatience or the appearance of being worldly-wise. The doctor must not be misled into believing that the patient has acquired a certain level of sex education from school, but must patiently find out what the patient needs to know.

The next case-history shows how a young girl asking aggressively for emergency contraception can be led to reveal her underlying feelings about sexual experience. In her case it was premature and in the wrong context, and to have simply responded to what she appeared to be asking for would have been to miss the real problem. The doctor here has to be especially careful to show a particular blend of concern and detachment with a prickly adolescent.

Hannah and her friends had made their presence felt in the clinic. The receptionist had experienced a great deal of sighing and impatient finger-tapping from Hannah as she completed the registration form. It was as if Hannah was sparing us a little of her precious time and we should not expect cooperation with the tedious clinic procedures.

Hannah and her friends proceeded to the waiting area, where their loud conversation and dancing to the radio were disturbing to other patients and clinic staff. Eventually Hannah was called in to my consulting room, where she sat chewing gum in her micro-skirt and skintight top. She said she was in a hurry and just needed 'the morning-after pill'. I felt myself being put in the position of just being a cipher, necessary to provide a prescription for this demanding patient. I wondered why Hannah needed to keep me at arm's length. I was aware that Hannah was using this casual attitude of disinterest as a defence, so decided to take on the role of physical doctoring and by this route contact the patient's feelings. I inquired about the date of Hannah's last period and why she felt the need for emergency contraception. Whilst I recorded the medical facts I made no comment or criticism, as I felt that the patient expected to be criticized for her behaviour. This approach seemed to give the young girl time to assess me and feel that it would be safe to expose her injured feelings. In a few moments a small, frightened girl emerged, who had had unprotected sex with an uncaring boyfriend.

She was 16 and had been pushed into physical sex by the boyfriend's friends, who had implied that there was something wrong with her, as 'He always has sex with girlfriends by now'. She had been afraid to ask him to use a condom, it had hurt a great deal and now she had an offensive green vaginal discharge. Hannah was truly terrified that she was anatomically abnormal – 'I think I have a tough hymen in the way' – and that she had contracted a venereal disease.

The doctor–patient relationship was now one of a concerned professional for an injured youngster. It was necessary to examine Hannah and when she was on the couch she was able to tell me that the friends who had brought her had told her of the terrors of examination and this was her reason for demanding emergency contraception and trying to keep the doctor at a distance. However, the examination was different from her expectations and she was able to ask basic anatomical questions. I gently took a swab as she was concerned about the boyfriend's apparent past sexual history of many partners and lack of condom usage.

Hannah was grateful for my concern and even listened attentively to an explanation of how to use post-coital contraception and its method of working. I noticed that the chewing gum had been consigned to the rubbish bin. Further contraception was offered and Hannah left with condoms, but it seemed that this patient would wait a while and be more discriminating about her next sexual encounter. She would be coming for a follow-up visit and more would be discussed about relationships, contraception, venereal disease and HIV infection. When she walked back into the waiting area the group of girlfriends clustered around Hannah and sensed a change in her. They all went downstairs in a more subdued manner.

Adolescence is a time for rebelling against the Establishment in any shape or form, including parents and doctors. Research has shown that this age group has the lowest rate of attendance at their GP's surgery and thus form a poor relationship with their family doctor (Obaid, 1992). They are embarking on a new stage of life and often wish to keep this away from their parents. Doctors can find them unapproachable when they attend clinics presenting a prickly exterior in dress, hairstyle and manner. It is important that they meet understanding in the consultation, and that their aggression is not met by the doctor's aggression.

THE DIFFICULT PATIENT

All the patients reported so far have had their discomforts and problems resolved to a greater or lesser extent. They have been able to accept a psychosomatic method of treatment and to understand when the doctor moved from physical to psychotherapeutic mode. The following case illustrates that the doctor cannot force this line of treatment on a patient who is determined to resist.

In a busy gynaecology outpatient clinic Caroline was preceded by a nurse bearing an extremely thick file of notes. I had a few moments to glance over the notes and realize that this patient had been under the hospital for some time, had many complaints and had been investigated by several different departments; she had also failed to keep appointments.

The patient who arrived in the consulting room was in her mid-thirties and looked untidy in a way that showed she took little care of her appearance. Her make-up was heavy and poorly applied and her clothes were shapeless and dull. She was polysymptomatic and sounded querulous. The symptoms which were relevant to her attendance at a gynaecology clinic were her painful and irregular periods and a profound disinterest in sex, although she expressed a desire to have a child. This patient was uncomfortable to be with: she was vague and it was difficult to obtain a history of her medical problems. In fact she was a 'difficult patient'. She had already been investigated, minor pathology had been found and oral treatment had been prescribed, but she had taken it for only a few days. I pointed out that the many doctors the patient had seen had done all that was possible. Maybe the patient was angry with herself or her husband and this anger seemed to be turned towards the hospital, the doctors and the treatment. The patient had a disconcerting way at this juncture of trying to charm me and arguing that she really needed treatment. She had stopped the hormonal treatment given by the previous doctor, as she had developed unlikely symptoms on it. I felt a need to get rid of this difficult patient as soon as possible, so prescribed a slightly modified course of hormones and made an appointment to see her in three months.

At the next visit Caroline had not bothered to take the new treatment at all although she still had the same complaints. I acknowledged that this form of physical treatment was being rejected. Previously the patient and her husband had been referred for psychosexual counselling as their relationship was so poor, but they had not kept the appointment. I remarked that maybe the physical problems relating to her female parts were partly due to her sexual frustrations and counselling would help. The patient stood up and said, 'You're blaming it on my nerves aren't you? Doctors have tried to say that before.' She gathered her things together and noisily left the clinic.

This consultation left me feeling a failure. As healers the whole purpose of our work is to help relieve physical and psychological discomfort. The case of Caroline demonstrates that the 'healing bond' is a process that requires the participation of doctor and patient. However enthusiastic the doctor is to do her job, she is bound to fail if the patient will not accept treatment. I had seen the rejection of physical treatment by the patient and had tried to change roles to a psychotherapeutic mode. Maybe the moment of change was presented to the patient at the wrong stage of her treatment when her anger at herself and her painful childless state was too intense. The disappointment and anger were thrown firmly on to me. I felt relief that I would not see this 'difficult patient' again, but sadness for the patient who could not walk away from her own pain.

CONCLUSION

These cases demonstrate the diversity of the work in family planning, gynaecology and psychosexual clinics. It is still a sad fact that medical students and doctors are taught the scientific facts associated with the prescribing of contraceptives, but they are not taught the communication skills which are necessary in this delicate, personal field of medicine. At present the patient can choose whether she attends her general practitioner or her community-based family planning clinic. In the financially motivated rationalization of health care provision several community-based family planning clinics have been closed, with the rationale that this facility is available at the GP's surgery. Many GPs who became principals prior to the GP training scheme have no postgraduate training or qualification in family planning. Others do not wish to offer this service to their patients as they feel it would bring embarrassment and difficulty in their ongoing relationship with the patient as their family doctor.

Some patients do not feel comfortable in approaching their GP for family planning advice or with an unwanted pregnancy. Attendance at a community-based clinic or a charitable organization such as the Brook Advisory Centre offers a degree of anonymity and confidentiality to the patient. The patients who live outside a large conurbation may well have less choice of clinics available to them. They feel that attending their local doctor or rural clinic will be far from anonymous and everyone will know their business. Alternatively some patients seek help from their GP for a psychosexual difficulty as they are confident that it is an advantage for the doctor to know them and their family. When the problem is resolved the patient feels able to attend the GP's surgery with purely physical problems. When this happens the patient puts the doctor back into the role of a physical doctor and never mentions the sexual difficulty again.

So we see that even before the doctor and patient meet there are several factors to take into consideration. At this stage the patient is attempting to choose between a family doctor who knows her medical history or a clinic doctor who is well trained in this field but does not know the patient. In the case of the psychosexual problem clinic the patient has often requested help from the family doctor, who has referred her on to the specialist. This step may be too great for the patient and she might never attend the appointment as she feels rejected by or too huge a problem for the family doctor. The referral to a psychosexual clinic is a very important stage in seeking help and requires sensitive handling by the general practitioner or the consultant concerned. Referring doctors need to convey to their patients how confident they feel about the suitability of the problem for referral. They need to know the qualifications and method of work of the particular psychosexual specialist, so that they can briefly explain to the patient what to expect at the clinic. Both time and National Health Service funds can be wasted by an inappropriate referral of a patient who was expecting a different way of working with his or her problem, for example a patient might be expecting a behaviourist approach to a psychosexual problem but experience a psychotherapeutic approach.

The psychosexual clinic might be held in a hospital or family planning clinic or even in a general practitioner's surgery, so that the patient will feel comfortable to a greater or lesser extent whilst waiting to see the doctor. A man, for example, might be distressed by a waiting area which is full of women patients and overt family planning posters and leaflets. If he is suffering from impotence he might feel that his problem is unusual and specific to him, when the rest of the community needs to restrict their reproductive capabilities. In this same way a frigid woman might be horrified by finding that her doctor is male, and unable to open up to him for therapy.

In a perfect world the doctor would have no preconceived ideas about the patient, but he or she can behave disruptively in the waiting area, and comments by receptionists and nurses will influence the doctor. When there is a referral letter the doctor is in receipt of another doctor's feelings about the patient and must find out what the patient feels is the problem, rather than give the label supplied by the referring doctor.

It is certainly more fruitful to study the doctor–patient relationship as it develops and changes during the consultation than to take the patient's history. The passive man seeking a reason for his impotence was able to understand his attitude to women when it was illustrated by the doctor–patient relationship. However, it is vital for him to accept the interpretation of this relationship and use it to alter his attitude and behaviour in his personal relationships. There was a point at which he accepted responsibility for his own actions and became potent.

The need for a patient to accept this responsibility and not expect the doctor to do all the work in reaching a 'cure' was also shown in the case of the 'injured patient'. Anthea could not use her vagina when it was still an injured part belonging to the doctors and nurses who had caused her so much pain. Her childlike fear in the relationship with the doctor in the family planning clinic needed interpretation before she could mature to the stage when she accepted her vagina to use as she desired.

There are patients who present their problems in the family planning or psychosexual clinic but expect the doctor to 'cure' them without any participation on their part. Sometimes a frigid woman will not look at her reasons for withholding herself both in her relationship with the doctor and with her sexual partner. She will constantly ask for surgery, so that someone else is taking the responsibility for physically opening her up. She makes the doctor feel as hopeless as she makes her partner feel. The doctor can work hard at interpretations for many weeks and then realize that there is no progress. The rate of change during treatment is totally patient-led; the doctor cannot speed this up. In the same way treatment cannot be forced on to the non-compliant patient, as illustrated by the last case-study.

There is the difficulty of finding the right point at which to stop treatment. Caroline chose to end her own treatment by storming out of the clinic. The end-point for treatment could be drawn on a graph with Caroline and her final exit at one end to long-term patients at the other end. In-between would be patients working at whatever rate they are able to use their therapy. Some cases take all the healer has to offer them, and even when the doctor feels that there is no chance of any further change and suggests the end of treatment the patient will not accept this and pleads for another appointment. This is part of the patient's inability to take responsibility for her own condition and her continuing dependence on the doctor. We saw in Ella's case that I was put into the role of a caring mother to replace Ella's neglectful mother and saw Ella for many months. Eventually this doctor–patient relationship changed as Ella accepted adulthood and reached the end of treatment.

It has been noted that cases in which the patient puts the doctor in the role of a mother figure or protector often lead to longer treatment than is usual. This is especially noticeable when seeing an adult who has been abused as a child. The patient needs the doctor to be a better, more concerned mother than her own mother. In contrast to this situation a doctor may feel that good interpretations have been made of the doctor–patient interaction during the consultation, only to find that the patient fails to attend the next appointment. When sexual happiness is achieved or regained the patient may consider that this is a private part of her life and no longer wants to share her feelings with the doctor. The doctor is left uncertain as to whether the patient derived enough from the consultation to feel cured and no longer needs the doctor. Alternatively the patient might be rejecting the form of treatment offered by the doctor, so the termination of this doctor–patient bond is patient-led. The doctor and patient have to define the delicate point at which sufficient work has been done for them to let go of each other; and, as illustrated, this varies greatly between cases.

REFERENCES

Conway, M., Bolt, S., Cooper, E., Gibbs, J., Howell, D., Thoms, M. and Yorstan, J. (1989) 'Long-term Psychosexual Problems following Termination of Pregnancy', *Journal of the Institute of Psychosexual Medicine*, 36: 13–19.

Lincoln, R. and Thexton, R. (1979) 'Patients Presenting with Non-Ejaculation', *British Journal of Sexual Medicine*, 6: 55–6.

Obaid, M. (1992) 'Dealing Sensitively with Teenage Pregnancy', unpublished paper given at teenage pregnancy conference in Cardiff, April.

Name index

References are to author and date of publication. Full details of publications should be found in the bibliography at the end of the chapter in which the references are found.

Subject index